Coaches' Guide to Enhancing Recovery in Athletes:

A Multidimensional Approach to Developing a "Performance Lifestyle"

Ian Jeffreys

COACHES CHOICE™

ISBN: 978-1-58518-677-8
Library of Congress Control Number: 2008925083
Cover design: Studio J Art & Design
Book layout: Studio J Art & Design
Front cover photo: ©EFE/ZUMA Press

Coaches Choice
P.O. Box 1828
Monterey, CA 93942
www.coacheschoice.com

Dedication

For Cath and James

Acknowledgments

To my wife, Catherine, and son, James. Without their support this text would not have been possible. Your love and support are the foundation for my own Performance Lifestyle.

To Peter Ashcroft for his help in producing the photographs.

To my father and mother, who instilled in me a passion for learning and sports, without which I would not have been able to pursue this great profession.

To all the staff at Coaches Choice, for their support through the production of the book.

Foreword

Ian Jeffreys' work builds a foundation from which all athletes can develop and optimize recovery strategies. The initial chapter of the text explains the fitness-fatigue relationship, which is paramount in the understanding of training theory. The interesting perspective of this chapter is that it looks at the multiple domains that the fitness-fatigue concept impacts. From this point, the text makes a strong argument for methods of removing fatigue, while maintaining the fitness that has been developed through training. After providing comprehensive coverage of these concepts, Jeffreys establishes a strong argument for the multilateral approach to dealing with recovery.

Traditionally, many coaches and authors think of recovery in a one-dimensional way that centers on the actual training plan. Jeffreys takes the concept of recovery to another level in the second part of this exciting text. He develops and explains the seven pillars from which to develop a lifestyle aimed at maximizing athletic performance. Conceptually, the seven pillars integrate the psychological and physiological needs of the athlete into a comprehensive plan that any coach or athlete can easily incorporate into his own training practices. The seven pillars of a high-performance lifestyle expand upon the current concepts in recovery theory and give practical guidelines from which to elevate performance to optimal levels.

This book is truly a groundbreaking text that will offer the coaching professional practical information that he can immediately integrate into his training practices. Ian Jeffreys take recovery theory to a new level, one that allows the coach to approach the athletes' needs on many fronts and culminates with the development of optimal performance.

—G. Gregory Haff, Ph.D., C.S.C.S.*D, FNSCA
Department of Human Performance and Applied Exercise Science
Division of Exercise Physiology
West Virginia University School of Medicine

Contents

Introduction

"There is nothing more powerful than an idea whose time has come."

—Victor Hugo

In today's competitive sports world, athletes are always after an edge over the opposition. They train longer, they train harder, they use any new system that may give them an edge, yet they consistently overlook an area that can definitely give them an edge—recovery. No matter how effectively athletes train, the simple fact is that a lack of recovery will hinder performance. Track and field athletes have long recognized the need to taper for major performances, and few of these athletes today even think of competing without a tapering period. In essence, tapering is simply a system to allow for full levels of recovery, and hence super-compensation. At this time, recovery is given a high priority, yet recovery is often overlooked during day-to-day training. In the development of training programs, recovery receives nowhere near the attention devoted to training. However, this thinking is severely flawed, as recovery is fundamental to optimal performance and should receive equal attention.

Underrecovery will always compromise performance, and to be effective any performance-enhancement program must ensure that recovery is as well-planned and programmed as the athlete's training. Indeed, the use of effective recovery strategies may be one of the most potent tools in a coach's arsenal. A well-recovered athlete can perform at a higher level, both in training and competition, thereby ensuring that the high-quality work needed for adaptation is completed. Similarly, with the use of effective recovery strategies, athletes are able to recover more rapidly and more effectively, allowing for more effective super-compensation and, hence, training progress. A well-planned recovery program is clearly fundamental to any athlete's development program and may be the next frontier in sports training.

What will become clear in the book is that an effective recovery program must be both multidimensional and individualized if it is to be optimally effective. The Performance Lifestyle provides athletes and coaches with a framework from which to construct effective recovery strategies that can be individualized for all athletes and situations. A unique feature of the Performance Lifestyle approach to enhancing recovery and performance is its multidimensional nature, which integrates research from a wide variety of performance areas into a holistic whole. This process focuses on the creation and management of energy in all aspects of the athlete's life. Today's athlete lives in a world where demands upon time and energy are at their greatest. In addition to being athletes, they play other roles such as student, partner, friend, etc., all of which create energy requirements above and beyond those of the athletic realm. The Performance Lifestyle looks at an athlete as a whole person, not simply as an athlete. Every facet of an athlete's life has the capacity to either create or destroy energy, and contribute to the overall stress levels of the athlete, and subsequently the levels of both recovery and performance.

While traditional approaches to training focus simply on the physical stressors of training, the Performance Lifestyle provides a multidimensional approach, which is vital in achieving optimal recovery levels. All stress, regardless of whether it originates from the training program or from any other aspect of the athlete's life, such as schoolwork, money issues, marital problems, etc., affects the whole person. By taking a multidimensional approach, the athlete and coach are able to control overall stress levels, not simply physical stress levels. They are then able to deal proactively with each individual source, contributing to effective energy management and enhanced overall recovery.

The Performance Lifestyle provides coaches and athletes with a structure around which to build individualized and multidimensional recovery strategies that both optimize recovery and maximize performance levels. They will also build skills with which to optimize performance both within and outside the athletic arena. The multidimensional approach will be the preferred system of recovery in the future, and the Performance Lifestyle provides coaches and athletes with the tools to initiate this in their programs starting today.

Part I: The Multidimensional Nature of Recovery in Athletes

1

The Nature of Fitness, Fatigue, and Recovery

"Optimal performance is only achievable if athletes recover after competition and optimally balance training stress and adequate recovery."

—Kellmann, 2002

Coaches and athletes are constantly trying to improve athletes' levels of performance. To facilitate this effort, a great body of research has been conducted exploring the best methods of enhancing performance through training. Modern athletes are undertaking ever more sophisticated systems of training that involve strength and conditioning as well as traditional sport-specific training, both of which are now acknowledged as key aspects of an athlete's performance-enhancement program. While these systems are meticulously planned, one key area remains in which many training programs fall down—and that is recovery. This oversight is unfortunate, as without adequate recovery, performance levels will always be compromised.

The Need for a Recovery Focus

The aim of any training program is to enhance athletic performance, yet athletes will only achieve optimal performance if a balance exists between training and recovery, regardless of how sophisticated the training system is. While training programs are meticulously planned to provide the required stimuli to enhance performance, with coaches often spending hours attempting to construct the "perfect training program," recovery is often neglected. For training to be optimally effective, it needs to be subjected to the same levels of planning and programming as the training stimulus. The planning and programming of recovery may be the key area that can elevate athletic performance to another level. It must always be remembered that optimal training progress requires a careful balance between stimulation and recovery, and if recovery is not sufficient, then training progress will be adversely affected.

The perfect training program is simply not possible without taking into account the factors that will affect recovery, which requires a focus on both the training program itself and on the factors that affect an athlete's response to the training, including an athlete's perception of the training and his response to the stimulus provided. Addressing individual needs for recovery in the training program is a key step in providing for the optimal training response. Despite this clear need for recovery, it remains an underaddressed element in many programs.

This lack of emphasis on recovery is also evident in the sport-science literature. A simple search of any performance journal will reveal how little work is carried out on recovery, yet the simple fact remains that recovery is a potent tool for any athlete wishing to enhance his performance.

Underrecovery and Overtraining

One area of work that has received some attention over the years has been the issue of overtraining, which has long been seen as a problem for many athletes. Overtraining syndrome is now commonly accepted in the sport-science literature and is evident at a wide range of levels, not just with elite athletes. Overtraining can be looked at as an imbalance between training stress and recovery and is normally characterized by a plateau or decrement in performance. Athletes normally diagnosed with overtraining syndrome demonstrate one or more of a number of characteristics, which can include the following:

- An increased resting heart rate
- A loss of body weight
- A decrease in appetite
- Restlessness or irritability
- Muscle soreness that lasts more than 24 hours
- Poorer work economy and increased submaximal heart rate
- An increase in illness
- A decrease in performance
- A lack of desire in training or competing

An interesting feature of these characteristics is that they are multidimensional in nature. For example, while a loss of body weight is a physical indicator, a decrease in desire in training or competition is a psychological indicator, and restlessness and irritability are emotional indicators. In this way, psychological and emotional indicators can be identified along with the physical, and the effects of overtraining are likely to manifest themselves in different ways in different individuals. Similarly, the causes of what is commonly termed "overtraining syndrome" will differ among individuals. Each athlete will have his own unique ability to cope with various stressors, and therefore a single-dimension approach will never be optimal with all athletes. A multidimensional approach is fundamental to optimally addressing recovery. Additionally, the approach needs to be individualized to the precise requirements of each athlete. This multidimensional and individualized approach is the foundation of the Performance Lifestyle's philosophy of recovery enhancement.

Overtraining or Underrecovery?

While the term "overtraining" has been accepted in the sport science literature, in terms of enhancing recovery, this term may actually cloud some key issues revolving around whether the symptoms of overtraining syndrome are always due to excessive training. In some cases, excessive training may be the cause, but in many other cases the athlete simply hasn't recovered from the total stresses imposed on him, of which physical stresses are only one. Some athletes are able to cope with a given training load at one given time, yet show the symptoms of "overtraining" with the same training load at another. While this scenario may at first appear contradictory, especially if a single-dimension approach is taken (e.g., physical), a look at the athlete as a whole (the multidimensional approach) may shed light on the issue. Perhaps when he experienced the same load for a second time he was experiencing stresses in his personal life, such as the break-up of a relationship. In this case, the training stresses, superimposed on the life stresses, may have exceeded the stress capacity of the athlete—hence the appearance of symptoms traditionally associated with overtraining.

Given this need for a multidimensional approach to looking at stress and recovery, the Performance Lifestyle utilizes the term "underrecovery" rather than "overtraining." Underrecovery can be looked at as an imbalance between total stress and total recovery. This term better reflects the multidimensional approach needed to tackle recovery, but also widens the coach's focus and provides more strategies to deal with individual athletes. While the characteristics of overtraining listed earlier have been linked to what is commonly termed "overtraining," they can also all be attributed to underrecovery.

The Implications of the Underrecovery Approach

At first, this change in focus may appear to be a simple change in terminology. However, when looked at more closely, this approach actually produces significant shifts in the way the performance issues are examined. By its very nature, the term overtraining suggests that the problems are with the training program. This fact alone is a problem, as very often the training program is written by the coach, and so the athlete feels unable to have an impact on the problem. Additionally, if underperformance is attributed to overtraining, then it implicates a physical solution, normally a reduction or change in training load. The reality is that the problem is likely far more complex than what can be explained by a simple physical model. In reality, a wide variety of factors can affect the athlete's performance, and these factors will often involve psychological or emotional issues, in addition to any physical issues. Additionally, performance issues may be caused by factors outside of the athletic arena. Dealing with these types of issues requires a radical new approach, one that is provided by the Performance Lifestyle. By focusing on the multidimensional nature of underrecovery, the point of emphasis can be changed from a completely coach-orientated approach (concerned solely with training-program design and the planning of total training loads, etc.) to a shared coach-and-athlete approach, with both able to initiate individualized recovery programs.

The Fitness-Fatigue Theory—The Basis of Performance Lifestyle Training

In terms of looking at overall training stresses and the requirements for recovery, an important step is to look at the effects of a training session on an athlete. Doing so will provide an important insight into the need for recovery and the specific requirements for recovery. According to the fitness-fatigue theory proposed by Vladimir Zatziorsky (1995), any training session has two distinct effects on the body (Figure 1-1). One is a potentiation effect, or an enhancement of performance capacity, and the other is a fatiguing effect on the body. The relative effects of these components will depend upon the nature of the training stressor and the athlete's capacity to cope with the stimulus.

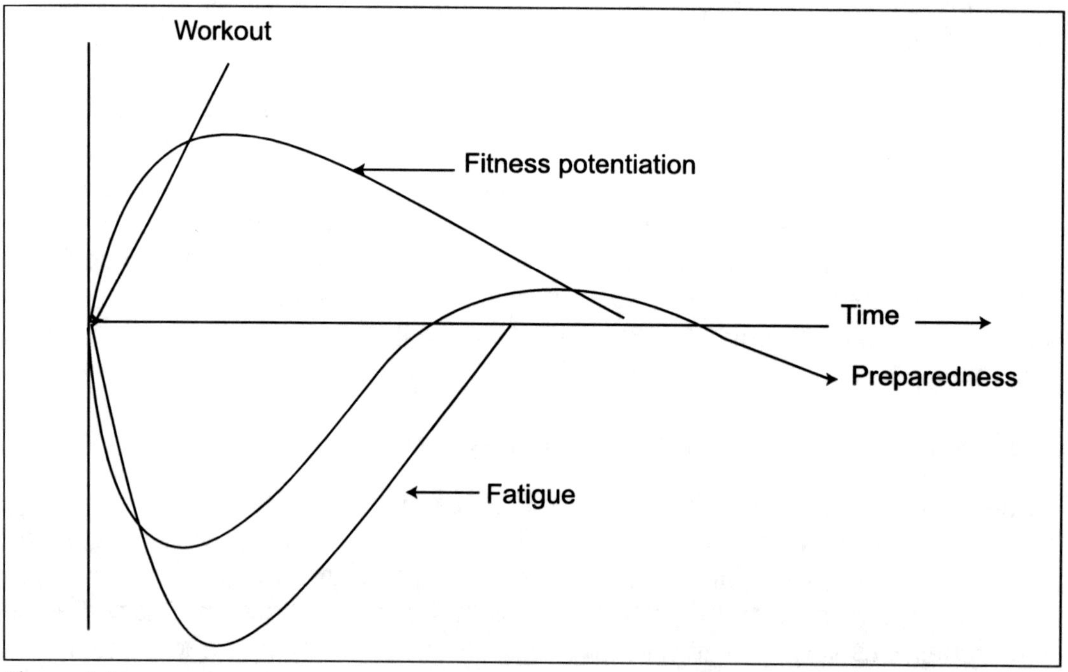

Figure 1-1

The potentiation effect involves an enhancement of performance. The training session will enhance the athlete's performance in the variable trained. For example, a speed-training session will enhance the athlete's running speed. However, immediately after the training session, despite this potentiation, the athlete's performance capacity will initially decline. Therefore, the athlete undertaking the speed session will probably run slower after the session than he did before. This performance decline is due to the impact of fatigue. In the short term, despite the training providing a potentiation effect, actual performance will decline due to fatigue.

A look at the performance level shows that in the period after a training session, an athlete's preparedness or performance will actually deteriorate, because the fatiguing elements of a workout are greater than the potentiation effects. However, as recovery proceeds, performance levels gradually increase as recovery from fatigue occurs. At this time, the body starts to super-compensate and increase performance capacity. The potentiation effects of the session allow for this super-compensation, the amount of which will depend upon the nature of potentiation, the nature of fatigue, and the nature of recovery. Training stress must be of sufficient quality to provide for optimal potentiation, and quality training is a vital part of an athlete's program. However, the full effects of the potentiating potential of training will never be experienced unless recovery is optimally addressed.

Optimizing the effects of recovery through a Performance Lifestyle approach can both minimize the effects of fatigue and maximize the levels of recovery—resulting in higher levels of super-compensation. This super-compensation is fundamental to enhancing performance through training, but must be seen to rely on the recovery side of the equation as well as on the training side. All too often, the recovery side of the equation is forgotten, resulting in less than optimal training progress.

The relative impact of potentiation and fatigue will be directly related not only to the actual training stimulus provided, but also to the athlete's ability to cope with these stressors at that particular time. Again, the importance of looking at both sides of the fitness-fatigue theory must be emphasized, and both athlete and coach must understand why a multidimensional approach is the only way to achieve optimal performance.

Aspects of the training stimulus will include the type of stressor (e.g., a strength-training session, a speed session), the intensity of the session, and the duration of the session. These aspects taken together will affect the overall nature of the stress, and their subsequent effect on potentiation, fatigue, and subsequent performance.

However, the training stimulus must never be seen in isolation, and instead must be directly related to the athlete's abilities at the time of training. The overall effect of the training will be directly related to the athlete's ability to cope with the training stimulus and his subsequent recovery ability. These training stresses will be superimposed on the athlete's current condition and capacity, and the coach needs to be aware of this situation when allocating the training load.

To ensure optimal performance, a coach clearly needs to ensure that the potentiation effects of a training program provide for super-compensation while attempting to offset the effects of fatigue via a well-planned proactive recovery program. This approach is aimed at minimizing both the duration and the extent of the fatiguing effects, allowing for more rapid super-compensation and ultimately the ability to cope effectively with the increased loads required at higher levels of performance. This capacity will depend upon a large number of interrelated factors, such as training status, general health, nutritional quality, sleep status, recovery from previous sessions, etc. These factors are addressed in detail within the pillars of the Performance Lifestyle (refer to Chapters 4 through 10).

Unfortunately, in many cases a response to a deterioration in performance is to increase the workload, a response that shows a lack of understanding of the fitness-fatigue theory. While this response may be prudent in some circumstances, in many it will simply exacerbate the problem, a problem that is often caused by underrecovery rather than a lack of stimulus. It is vital to keep in mind that if athletes have not recovered, they simply cannot work to their full capacity. A key to the Performance Lifestyle approach is that it looks at ways of making training more productive by training smart while providing for regeneration and recovery on a multidimensional basis. Recovery must be given the same importance as the training load in the planning process and must become a part of a Performance Lifestyle, an approach that is capable of enhancing recovery all day, every day.

The Nature of Fitness

The fitness-fatigue model introduced the term fitness, but an important aspect of fully utilizing the Performance Lifestyle approach to enhancing recovery and performance is more carefully considering the nature of fitness. Fitness is normally associated with physical fitness. However, physical fitness alone cannot accurately predict sports performance or subsequent recovery. Instead, fitness needs to be looked at from a multidimensional perspective, and this wider perspective is fundamental to the successful application of the Performance Lifestyle approach. Fitness and recovery can be seen to exist in three domains, with the degree of fitness and recovery dependent upon the complex inter-relationships and cybernetic links among these domains. The domains, which are represented in Figure 1-2, are as follows:

- The physical domain
- The psychological domain
- The emotional domain

The Physical Domain

This domain is most commonly associated with fitness, and involves elements such as speed, strength, and power. Physical training is, quite rightly, an integral part of any athlete's program. A huge amount of information exists in terms of utilizing the best training techniques and programs to develop sport-specific fitness. This information provides an excellent knowledge base upon which to build effective training programs. However, as has already been explained, recovery is an essential part of any training program, and the Performance Lifestyle focuses on the balance between training and recovery and utilizes strategies to enhance physical recovery.

The Psychological Domain

Peak athletic performance is not possible without effective performance in the psychological domain. Aspects such as confidence and mental toughness are generally regarded as essential elements of elite performance. Similarly, effective recovery can be compromised unless psychological capacity and recovery are developed. Developing mental capacities such as confidence, anxiety control, and relaxation is an important element of the Performance Lifestyle approach, together with strategies to enhance psychological recovery.

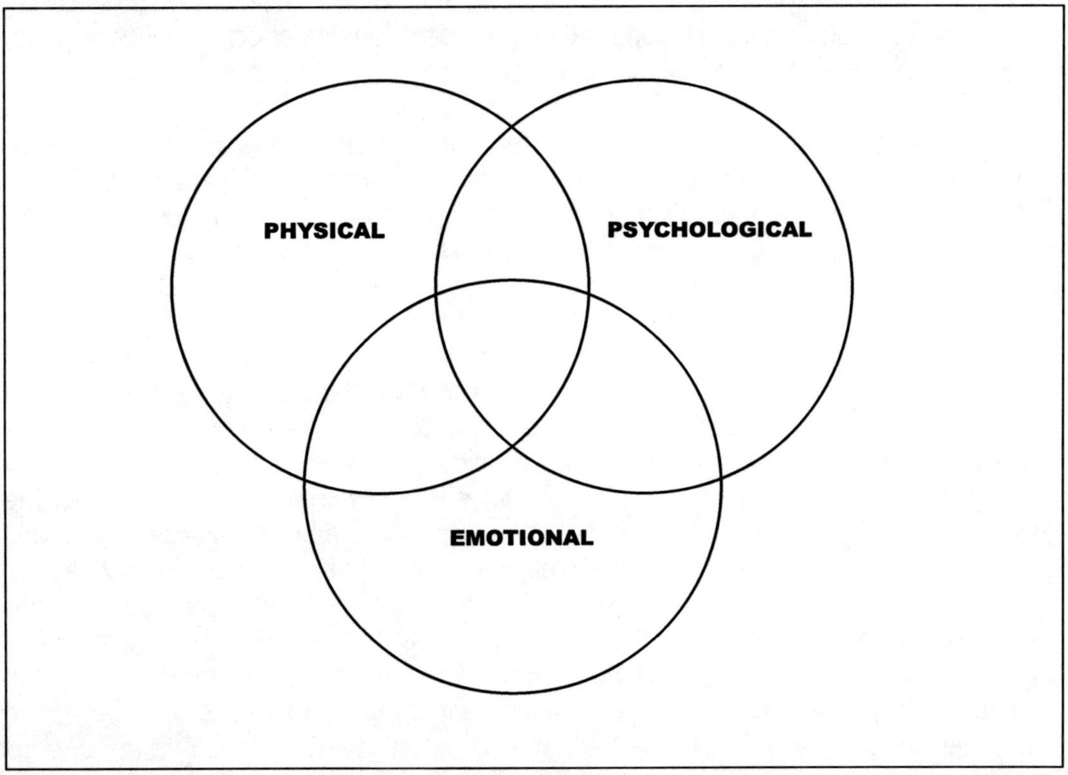

Figure 1-2

The Emotional Domain

The emotional domain is possibly the strongest of the domains, and an emotionally healthy athlete has a great capacity for training and recovery. However, this aspect of fitness can be eroded rapidly and needs to be constantly monitored and developed. An athlete's mind is active throughout each day, generating thoughts and feelings at all times. The way an athlete thinks and feels about something is often based upon his belief systems. Together, these beliefs create moods and feelings, which have the capacity to either energize or de-energize, and can significantly affect both performance and recovery. To capitalize on this capacity, developing the emotionally intelligent athlete is a fundamental part of the Performance Lifestyle program. This domain requires a focus on developing the emotional fitness that is required for elite performance, as well as optimal recovery. Emotional fitness is based on emotional intelligence and involves self-awareness and control, together with social awareness and control. Creating a positive emotional environment is one of the key elements of the Performance Lifestyle.

The Interrelationship of the Domains

While it is often easy to classify stress and recovery into one of the three domains, the effects are not so easy to classify. Human beings have needs in the three major fitness domains–physical, psychological and, emotional. The degree to which these needs are met, and the unique capability of the athlete in each domain, affect the overall quality of life. Similarly, athletes have specific requirements and capabilities within each domain.

Athletic performance is dependent upon the interrelationships among many factors, and total fitness must therefore be seen as multidimensional in nature, with each domain having the ability to both affect performance and influence recovery. Research is also highlighting the close relationship between performance in each of the different domains. For example, an athlete may be having problems with his relationship with his partner, and while this situation is easy to classify initially as emotional stress, it may cause negative feelings, such as guilt, depression, etc. Despite this problem being emotional in nature, it will also have the capacity to drain physical resources and cause psychological fatigue, both of which can inhibit recovery and subsequent performance. In this way, the emotional problem can manifest itself in all of the fitness domains. The capacities and states in one domain will clearly affect the capacity and states in the other domains. Developing the athlete requires developing performance in all domains. When all domains are not addressed, a potential weak link is created that can hinder both recovery and performance. Similarly, recovery strategies depend upon the interaction of all domains of fitness, further strengthening the need for a multidimensional approach that addresses all three domains. Given the complexity of these interrelationships, it is clear that these factors will vary from individual to individual. A key to the Performance Lifestyle approach is that the optimal recovery strategies need to be individualized to each athlete's specific needs.

The Nature of Fatigue

Just as the fitness-fatigue theory involves the concept of fitness, it also involves the concept of fatigue. When planning any recovery program, it is important to understand the nature of fatigue. Just as fitness has been shown to be multidimensional, involving performance in the three major fitness domains, fatigue similarly occurs in these three domains (Figure 1-3). The type and degree of fatigue is dependent upon the nature of the stressors experienced and the athlete's capacity in each domain.

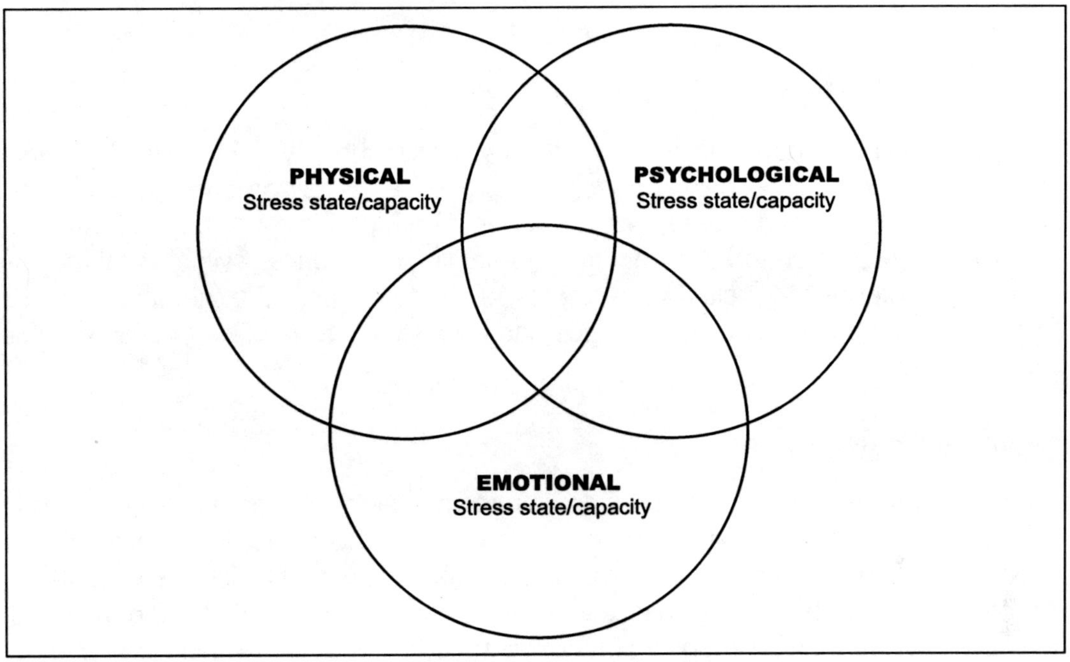

Figure 1-3

Physical Fatigue

Physical fatigue is the type of fatigue most often associated with training activities. Just as training effects are specific to the training stimulus, the type of physical fatigue is dependent upon the type of activity undertaken. In general, three main types of physical fatigue can be identified:

- *Physiological fatigue*: This type of physical fatigue is associated with the energy-producing capacity of the body. Physiological fatigue can result from a reduction in the body's energy stores (including glycogen, creatine phosphate, etc.) and from the creation of metabolic by-products that hinder performance, such as the build-up of lactic acid. Physiological fatigue is closely associated with activities involving long durations, such as distance running, and intermittent activities lasting for long durations, such as soccer.

- *Neural fatigue*: This type of physical fatigue is associated with a reduction in the contraction ability of the neuromuscular system. Far less is known about the exact causes of neural fatigue, but factors such as depletion of neurotransmitters have a significant effect on performance. Neural fatigue is especially associated with high-intensity activities such as sprinting, weight lifting, etc.
- *Tissue damage*: This type of physical fatigue is associated with trauma to the tissues, such as that caused by physical contact and eccentric muscle actions. This factor is especially important in sports that involve physical contact, such as football, rugby, etc., as well as training activities that involve intense eccentric activities, such as plyometrics.

Psychological Fatigue

Fatigue occurs in the psychological domain as well as in the physical domain. Elements such as monotony, boredom, and lack of confidence can all produce psychological fatigue in an athlete, and thereby negatively affect both performance and recovery. For example, an intense period of competition or training can induce psychological fatigue, due to the intense psychological pressures of these periods. Coaches and athletes need to be aware of psychological fatigue and have strategies in place to deal with this phenomenon.

Emotional Fatigue

Emotions provide for a very powerful domain in an athlete's performance. Emotionally healthy athletes have a massive capacity for training, and conversely, when emotional health is depleted, physical capacity can also decline. Everyone has felt elation, and the positive spill-over affects performance in all areas of a person's life. On the other hand, everyone has also all felt emotional lows, such as at the death of a close relative or friend, and experienced the negative effects such emotions have on all aspects of life. The quality of emotional management, the quality of personal relationships, and the ability to handle emotions will all affect the level of fatigue experienced in this domain. Athletes need to be able to recover emotionally, or they run the risk of setting up a long-term energy leak that can have serious long-term performance consequences.

The Nature of Recovery

Because fatigue occurs in a number of domains, recovery must also take a multidimensional approach. For optimal effectiveness, recovery needs to be a proactive process involving purposeful actions to enhance recovery. This process needs to occur in all three major domains—physical, psychological, and emotional. It is possible for an athlete to be in a good state of recovery in one domain but be underrecovered in one of the other domains. The net effect of this situation is that the athlete will be underperforming, as the lack of recovery in the one domain will hold back overall recovery and subsequent performance.

Time scales for recovery can also vary, with some aspects requiring a far greater period of recovery than others. Recovery from football, for example, will require a greater time than from basketball due to the greater physical fatigue caused by tissue damage, etc. Similarly, the effect of stressors can be immediate or delayed. For example, the effects of poor nutrition may not be immediately apparent and may take an extended period before their full effect is felt. The Performance Lifestyle provides a unique system that can provide for both short- and long-term recovery in all dimensions of fitness, and provides for the ideal long-term high-performance environment.

The Individual Nature of Recovery

Given the complex inter-relationships among the fitness domains and the unique levels of stress experienced by athletes, each individual will have his own requirements in terms of recovery. Similarly, individual preferences exist in terms of recovery strategies, and what works ideally for one athlete may not work effectively for another. This individualization of recovery at first presents a massive challenge to a coach, but the Performance Lifestyle is built around this individualization of recovery and encourages athletes to become aware of the nature of the stressors, their subsequent fatigue levels, and their preferred recovery strategies. In this way, individual strategies can be developed that address each athlete's unique stressors, with his own preferred systems providing for an individualized high-performance environment—a Performance Lifestyle.

The Additive Nature of Stressors

It must always be remembered that an athlete is a person, a unique psychosociophysiological system, and that he has a life away from athletics. All too often, coaches will forget this fact and not take into account the stressors that athletes are experiencing away from the athletic arena. In short, athletes must not be seen merely as physical beings. They are subjected to a range of stressors over and above those experienced within the training program on a daily basis. Stress itself can be seen as any factor that causes a deviation from the norm and can manifest itself in all three domains of fitness. Stress for athletes will include training and competition stress, but will also include non-training-related stressors. Aspects such as schoolwork, travel, and relationships all have the potential to become stressors for the athlete. Thus, training must never be seen in isolation, and other potential stressors must be taken into account when assessing an athlete's performance and planning training programs. Figure 1-4 demonstrates how the three domains of fatigue and stress have an accumulative effect on the body.

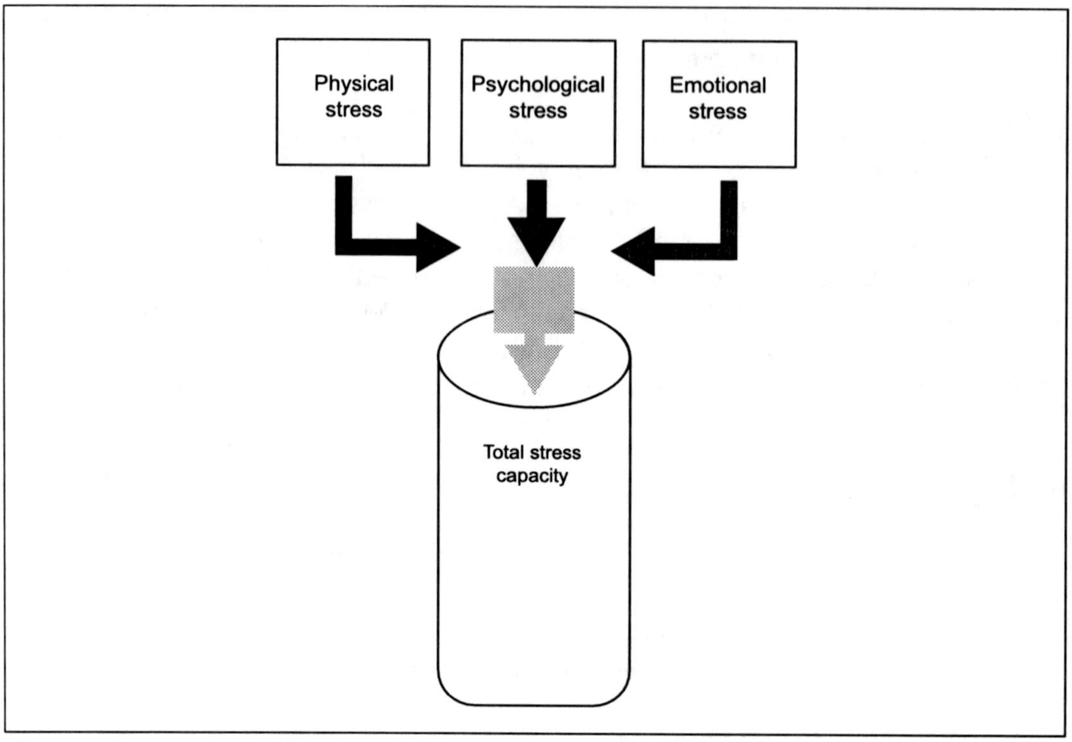

Figure 1-4

Figure 1-4 shows how all three domains of fitness can provide stress for the athlete, stress that all collects in the same melting pot. While stress is needed in all domains to develop performance, if at any time the stress exceeds the overall capacity, then it will undoubtedly have negative effects on recovery and performance. Additionally, stress from one domain can affect stress in other domains (e.g., at times of high physical stress, such as in training camps, an athlete my feel increasingly agitated and restless, indicating increased levels of psychological and emotional stress). Stress must never be seen in isolation, as a cybernetic link exists among all of the domains.

The long-term key for an athlete is to be able to build his overall capacity for stress, and that capacity must be developed in all three domains. At the same time, he needs to ensure that overall stress in each domain is controlled, so that sufficient overload is provided for enhanced performance, but without negatively affecting overall performance levels. This balance can be achieved by targeting training and then providing for appropriate regeneration activities, as will be outlined in Chapter 8. Similarly, athletes need to plan for appropriate high-stress situations, such as training camps, playoffs, examinations, etc. At times when stress levels will be higher, other activities will need to be reduced to ensure that the overall stress capacity is not exceeded. For example, during examination periods, physical training stress would need to be reduced to reflect this increase in psychological stress.

Summary

- Optimal performance is dependent upon effective recovery.
- Recovery needs to become central to any performance-enhancement program.
- By focusing on underrecovery rather that overtraining, the need for a multidimensional approach to recovery becomes evident.
- Fitness, fatigue, and recovery occur in three domains—physical, psychological, and emotional.
- Recovery needs to occur in all three domains to be optimally effective.
- Stress and fatigue will be highly individualized. Therefore, individualized recovery strategies are needed for optimal effectiveness.

2

A Multidimensional Approach to Recovery

"Health is a large word. It embraces not the body only, but the mind and spirit as well...and not today's pain or pleasure alone, but the whole being and outlook of a man."

—James H. West

Chapter 1 discussed the fact that fitness, fatigue, and subsequent recovery all occur in three domains. Similarly, overall fitness is subject to the complex inter-relationships among these domains. Therefore, optimal recovery can only be achieved if all three domains are addressed during the recovery process. Simply concentrating on one element of a recovery strategy, while better than doing nothing at all, cannot address all of the required areas of an overall recovery system. Clearly, any effective recovery program must take a multidimensional approach to this vital aspect of any training program. The Performance Lifestyle is an integrated, multidimensional program that addresses an athlete's unique individual needs across all domains, allowing for an individualized, multidimensional approach to recovery.

Performance and Recovery Through Managing Energy

The Performance Lifestyle is built around managing energy. All activities have the capacity to either build or expend energy within the body. As with any system, energy efficiency will be critical to optimal performance. Any energy efficiency campaign, regardless of the type of business, will try to minimize the energy expended in achieving the business aims, while also ensuring that sufficient stores of energy are available to allow the business to function to its optimal capacity. Additionally, it will ensure that no leaks of energy are contributing to inefficiency. In short, it aims to achieve optimal output at maximal energy efficiency, ensure energy stores are replenished to allow for repeated functions, and reduce energy leaks to maximize efficiency.

The Performance Lifestyle is built in the same way. It tries to ensure that through efficacious training, the athlete can develop all of the elements of performance that he will need to compete, without the expenditure of needless energy. At the same time, it ensures that energy stores are regenerated through the use of effective strategies such as sleep, nutrition, emotional regeneration, etc. It also works to identify and eradicate energy leaks, such as those caused by emotional issues, sleep problems, etc. In his groundbreaking book, *Flow*, Mihaly Csikszentmihalyi (2002) emphasizes how a person creates his quality of life and experiences by the way he invests his psychic energy (i.e., the attention that he gives different aspects of his life). He emphasizes that the investment of energy is within a person's control, and that appropriate energy investment is a vital tool in improving the quality of experience.

By utilizing this approach, energy expended is targeted at specific parameters, energy is regenerated through appropriate recovery strategies, and energy leaks are minimized. Athletes become energy efficient, leading to enhanced recovery and subsequent performance.

Recovery Through Building Capacity

An interesting aspect of recovery within the Performance Lifestyle is the need to build capacity, as outlined in Chapter 1. While looking at enhancing recovery through focusing on building capacity may at first seem strange, a close link exists between an athlete's capacity in each domain and his ability to recover. The greater the capacity to cope with the stressors placed on him, the less the overall fatigue that these stressors cause, and the greater the likelihood of recovery.

Capacity building is one of the key pillars of the Performance Lifestyle (refer to Chapter 8). Interestingly, capacity needs to be both multidimensional and specific, which again may seem contradictory at first glance. Simply stated, capacity needs to be built into all dimensions of fitness (multidimensional), but within each domain, capacity needs to be targeted at specific areas that are contributing to an athlete's lack of recovery.

A multidimensional approach to training is crucial for optimal performance. Athletes must not spend time building great capacity in one dimension at the expense of the other. Only by addressing all domains will they achieve full capacity, and hence full stress tolerance and recovery. Unfortunately, this multidimensional approach is seldom utilized in most training programs, where physical capacity is developed to a high degree, but with little or no work done to build psychological or emotional capacity. In these cases, athletes are often in great physical condition, yet fail to achieve their full potential due to their inability to cope with psychological pressure or emotional problems.

Similarly, this capacity can be specific within each domain. All of the domains involve a number of specific features. For example, the physical domain will involve elements such as strength, speed, and endurance, the psychological domain will include elements such as anxiety control and confidence, and the emotional domain will involve elements such as self-awareness, self-control, and social awareness. The capacity built must be related to the type of stress typically experienced, together with the athlete's current capacity. Training can then be targeted at the areas that will bring optimal results. Additionally, with targeted training, the overall stress load can be controlled, as time and energy are not wasted working on nonproductive areas. In this way, optimal results for a given training load can be achieved. Targeting also has the advantage of reducing the levels of nonproductive stress, or stress that adds to fatigue but brings a low level of benefit.

The Performance Lifestyle approach to recovery therefore requires athletes to build capacity into all of the fitness domains over time and address any weakness they have in each domain. By doing so, athletes will optimally increase their overall stress tolerance, ensuring that the stressors impact recovery to a lesser degree, thus facilitating faster recovery and greater performance.

Relate Stress to State

In addition to focusing on overall capacity, it is important that athletes note their current state within each domain. State can be likened to preparedness in the fitness-fatigue theory, a factor that will be in constant flux depending upon the relative effects of stress and recovery. They need to remember that they have an overall capacity for stress, and that it is related to the unique relationships among all domains. They will experience times when overall stress levels in some domains reach very high levels. In these situations, their actual "state" in these domains will decrease due to accumulated fatigue, reducing their ability to tolerate large amounts of additional stress from other domains. For example, during training camp, the physical stress will be great and the athletes' overall state will decrease due to high levels of fatigue. This situation requires that athletes proactively and appropriately increase their recovery activities. Additionally, it is important that they simultaneously try to reduce the amount of stress in the other domains. This time is not when an athlete should be planning a wedding, sitting for exams, or performing any other activities that will produce stress.

To facilitate this ability to react to recovery needs, a key pillar of the Performance Lifestyle is self-awareness (refer to Chapter 5). Self-awareness develops an athlete's ability to note his state in each domain, and allows him to both build appropriate targeted capacity and adjust stress loads at times when he notes a reduction in capacity in any domain.

Proactive Recovery

Hopefully, the need for an integrated recovery approach within a program is self-evident at this point. It cannot be stated too strongly that recovery needs to be an integral part of any athlete's program and has the capacity to greatly enhance any training program he is following. The approach recommended within the Performance Lifestyle is that an athlete takes a proactive approach to recovery, which involves monitoring the levels of fatigue and actively engaging in activities that can promote recovery in all domains. This active engagement is the key to proactive recovery, as it involves actively evaluating the current state and its effect on recovery. It also involves analyzing the effectiveness of various recovery strategies and then engaging in the preferred activities as required. Only in this way can an athlete take charge of his recovery actions and ensure that they are in line with his stress levels at any given time.

Passive and Active Recovery

Recovery activities are varied, and over time an athlete needs to develop his own preferred strategies. However, it is possible to classify recovery activities as either passive or active.

Passive activities involve aspects such as power naps, massage, and hydrotherapies. Despite being termed "passive," all of these techniques can be seen as proactive, as the athlete has the choice of how and when to use them. The key is for the athlete to identify activities that enhance his recovery ability (refer to Chapter 5). He will then be able to utilize these techniques however and whenever they are required.

Active recovery involves activities performed at a low level of exertion, all aimed at enhancing the body's recovery functions. Active recovery involves activities such as cool-downs and pool sessions. Like passive activities, these strategies need to be evaluated in terms of their effectiveness and then utilized proactively however and whenever they are needed. Chapter 8 outlines strategies and provides advice on when those strategies are most effective.

The Empowered Athlete and the Performance Lifestyle

Every day, athletes make hundreds of choices, both consciously and subconsciously, many of which will either directly or indirectly affect their recovery. Decisions such as when to go to bed, what leisure-time activities to pursue, and what to have for lunch will all potentially affect an athlete's level of recovery. Indeed, life can be seen as a sum total of the choices made. While a coach is able to directly affect what happens when the athlete is under his control (aspects such as the training program), the majority of recovery-based decisions lie with the athlete and occur away from the training arena. Athletes will often feel better when they are able to make choices, rather than be dictated to at all times. However, for optimal effectiveness, these choices need to be well-founded. It is important, therefore, that all athletes develop the knowledge base from which to make decisions that positively affect their recovery and subsequent performance. An effective education program should be a part of any performance-enhancement program, and an empowered athlete is therefore fundamental to the Performance Lifestyle approach.

The Empowered Athlete

To develop an effective Performance Lifestyle, athletes need to be empowered to make educated decisions. The empowered athlete has the knowledge and intelligence to make informed decisions about potential choices, together with the ability to put the knowledge into action via strategies and rituals. He also should possess the self-awareness to evaluate his capacities and the success of various strategies.

Aspects of the Empowered Athlete

An athlete-empowerment program should involve the following key strategies. Taken together, these four strategies allow for the individualized approach to performance and recovery, which is vital for optimal performance.

- The development of performance knowledge
- The development of self-awareness
- Awareness of strategies to put the knowledge into practice
- The motivation to take action

Knowledge is Power

The Performance Lifestyle approach to performance enhancement requires that the athletes take responsibility for the many choices they make on a daily basis. To do so, athletes need both the knowledge on which to base decisions and strategies to put the knowledge into practice. The Performance Lifestyle provides athletes with the required knowledge to set up an effective recovery program. Aspects such as what to eat, when to eat, what to do after a workout, and how to relax are all part of the knowledge required for a fully empowered athlete.

The Self-Aware Athlete

In an attempt to monitor the levels of recovery and stress, the athlete consistently needs to be able to answer key questions, including the following:

- How recovered am I?
- What stress am I experiencing?
- What is causing the stress?
- How is it affecting my performance?
- What recovery strategies work best for me?
- What recovery strategies should I be using at this time?

Because all of these answers will be specific to the individual, each athlete will need to come up with his own answers. Self-awareness is a key skill in all of the domains of fitness and recovery, and is the way in which the athlete can develop his ability to answer these key questions. Athletes who fail to notice key signs of underrecovery are unable to effectively undertake or evaluate activities that may enhance recovery. Self-awareness allows athletes to identify activities, thoughts, and habits that are draining energy. It also allows them to identify the effectiveness of the various strategies and rituals undertaken. Over time, athletes will be able to develop their own individualized strategies, which lie at the heart of the Performance Lifestyle.

To Know and Not Do is to Not Know

Despite the importance of knowledge, knowledge in itself is never effective. Knowledge only becomes a part of the Performance Lifestyle when put into action. The application of knowledge is what produces results. When knowledge is put into action, it is internalized, and only then is true knowledge evident. By putting the knowledge into action and monitoring the results, self-knowledge is developed. Self-knowledge is fundamental to the development of the individualized recovery strategies promoted by the Performance Lifestyle. This degree of self-knowledge is best learned through action, and all the information in the world will not be effective until it is put into action. The Performance Lifestyle utilizes the power of the ritual, a simple yet effective method by which knowledge can be translated into action (refer to Chapter 7).

Motivation Provides a Purpose

When actions required match an athlete's goals, then the likelihood of sustained action is maximized. A fundamental part of any factual education program must lie equally in the "why" as the "how." Athletes need to be made aware of why they should undertake certain activities and specifically how these activities will help them achieve their goals of better performance, especially when unfamiliar concepts are involved. In the pillars of the Performance Lifestyle outlined later in this book, strategies to enhance recovery in all of the domains of fitness are discussed. While some strategies, such as cooling down, may be self-evident to the athlete, others, such as emotional control, are more obtuse. Before these strategies are introduced, it is vital that their roles in total energy expenditure and recovery are fully understood by the athlete, and that appropriate implementation strategies are outlined. Once this foundation is available, the likelihood of athletes incorporating the strategies into their Performance Lifestyle is enhanced.

Summary

- Optimal recovery requires the management of energy.
- For optimal energy efficiency, an athlete needs to build his capacity in all domains of fitness.
- Capacity needs to be multidimensional and targeted at key weaknesses within each domain.
- Recovery needs to be proactive and involve active engagement with strategies that enhance recovery in all dimensions.
- The key to the individualization of recovery strategies is an empowered athlete.
- Athletes need to be empowered with knowledge, but also be given strategies by which this knowledge can be turned into actions.
- Rituals provide an ideal method by which recovery strategies can be put in place (refer to Chapter 7).

3

The Performance Lifestyle Model

"Life is the sum of all your choices."
—Albert Camus

The Performance Lifestyle model is based upon years of working with hundreds of athletes at all levels, and analysis of the wide-ranging factors that have affected their performance. It provides for the multidimensional and individualized approach outlined in the previous chapters. Within this system, empowered athletes are provided with the knowledge and tools to develop individualized rituals that lead to greater recovery and subsequent high-level performance. By addressing both the individualized and multidimensional natures of recovery, the Performance Lifestyle provides a powerful tool with which an athlete can develop his own recovery program.

The Performance Lifestyle is itself built around seven pillars, which, when taken together, address all aspects of a multidimensional integrated recovery system. Each pillar is important by itself, but when integrated with all of the other pillars, provides a powerful tool that enhances recovery in sports. Additionally, this system has a massive spill-over effect on performance, as it provides for an ideal environment in all three domains of fitness, which together provide the necessary conditions for optimal performance. The system itself can also be applied to life and can be used by any person wishing to enhance his performance in sport, business, or life.

Pillar 1—Identify and Act on Dreams

Unmet needs of any kind are a major drain on energy resources, and providing athletes with systems that help them address their key needs is a crucial element in energy management. Work on the *Flow* experience by Csikszentmihalyi (2002) demonstrates the relationships between optimal experience and clear goals, and how goals provide a framework around which to build an effective performance program. This pillar outlines the need for clear goals to ensure that athletes' energies are focused on achieving their identified dreams. This pillar helps athletes develop a clear roadmap toward their dreams, and describes how this goal can be achieved. Pillar 1 allows athletes to prepare an action plan to enable them to achieve their athletic dreams while also ensuring that they do not overlook activities that make life fulfilling. This pillar provides the focused, motivated approach that optimally utilizes energy and is vital for optimum performance.

Pillar 2—Develop Self-Awareness

Self-aware athletes are able to constantly monitor their performance and recovery levels and make appropriate adjustments in all of their fitness and recovery domains. This pillar outlines how awareness can be developed in all three domains, allowing athletes to identify their recovery levels, sources of stress, and recovery needs. It also enables them to evaluate various methods of enhancing recovery and develop systems that work for them. This process allows them to make the appropriate actions to enhance recovery and subsequent performance.

Pillar 3—The Power of Positive

A positive outlook is vital to both performance and recovery. Negative thoughts and beliefs can sap athletes of energy, reducing their overall capacity and hindering subsequent recovery. Positivity in all aspects of performance is vital to optimal performance. This pillar stresses the importance of a positive outlook on performance and recovery and outlines how it can be achieved.

Pillar 4—The Power of Rituals

Once self-awareness has been developed, it is vital that athletes initiate activities that directly address issues that are compromising recovery. Rituals are the preferred method of achieving optimal recovery in the Performance Lifestyle. Unlike self-discipline, which has a high energy requirement, rituals have low energy requirements, but are highly effective. Effective rituals are the backbone of the Performance Lifestyle and allow for optimum recovery with little energy expenditure. This pillar outlines how to set up effective rituals.

Pillar 5—Build Capacity and Regenerate

The need to build capacity in all domains has been consistently emphasized, as has the need for proactive recovery. This pillar of the Performance lifestyle model ensures that athletes are able to perform in each domain by building capacity and allowing subsequent regeneration. Athletes will build capacity in the three major domains of fitness—physical, psychological, and emotional—followed by regeneration and recovery. This pillar outlines effective strategies by which this outcome can be achieved.

Pillar 6—Quality Nutrition

Nutrition is vital for optimal recovery, ensuring that sufficient quality calories and nutrients are available in the correct quantities at the right time. This pillar outlines the keys to optimize health and recovery through engineered nutrition. It outlines strategies to design effective eating patterns that contribute to both optimum recovery and optimum performance.

Pillar 7—Quality Sleep

Sleep, both quantity and quality, is vital for recovery. This pillar outlines the keys to optimizing sleep and gives recommendations and strategies for ensuring that optimal sleep is achieved.

Part II: The Seven Pillars of the Performance Lifestyle

4

Pillar 1—Identify and Act on Dreams

"You can achieve anything you want in life if you have the courage to dream it, the intelligence to make a realistic plan, and the will to see the plan through to the end."
—Sidney A. Friedman

As outlined previously, the management of energy is a key principle for effective recovery. The quality of athletic performance and recovery will be very much influenced by the decisions athletes make on a daily basis, both large and small. It is important that athletes learn to devote energies to the activities that will be productive to their performances, and to ensure that energy-sapping activities are minimized. While this advice might appear relatively straightforward, it is vital that an athlete is able to identify such activities. Part of this ability will come from a clear view of what an athlete wants to achieve, together with the ability to build a clear pathway toward this goal. In this way, productive activities that contribute to the goals can be identified and promoted, while nonproductive activities can be identified and progressively removed from an athlete's life.

Additionally, it is important that athlete have clear goals away from the athletic arena and become aware of the activities that contribute to his personal happiness and fulfilment. Unfulfilled dreams and needs have the potential to be a massive drain on energy. Whenever people are unable to meet their deepest needs, it places a drain on their energy reserves, subsequently reducing levels of recovery and performance. Unfortunately, in the modern lifestyle where the requirements on time seem endless, people often fail to attend to their main needs, and this situation can last for days, weeks, months, or even years on end.

The Need for Clear Goals

What is required, both within and outside of athletics is a clear goal, together with a well-aligned pathway that identifies and meets needs on a regular basis. Goals allow people to see clearly where they want to get to, and creating a path to these goals can enhance the likelihood of them being achieved.

Csikszentmihalyi (2002), in his book entitled *Flow*, clearly emphasises the link between optimal experience and clear goals. "Flow" seems to happen most often when psychic energy is invested in realistic goals. This pursuit of a goal brings a level of order to an athlete's awareness, which is vital for optimal functioning. With the goal in place, the athlete can concentrate his attention on the task at hand. To achieve this state, goals need to be challenging yet attainable, continually moving an athlete forward. Additionally, the athlete needs feedback on whether the goal was attained. The type of this feedback can vary, but it is important that the athlete is aware of his progress toward the goal. Challenging yet attainable goals, which move an athlete forward toward a dream, engage the athlete's energy, yet provide regular success. This success develops a stronger, more confident self, as more psychic energy has been invested in goals he himself has chosen to pursue. This more confident self in turn contributes to a positive self-image that is vital to optimal performance and recovery (refer to Chapter 6).

To be optimally effective, it is essential that this plan addresses all needs, not merely those associated with athletics. While athletic goals may or not be the most important, it is vital that other needs are also identified and addressed. These goals could include career goals, the needs of family, individual interests, etc. By structuring life around meeting these goals, potential energy leaks can be reduced and optimal recovery is facilitated.

What Gets Measured Gets Done

A key aspect of many of the pillars of the Performance Lifestyle, including this first pillar, is the need for athletes to commit to writing things down. Writing things down greatly increases an individual's commitment to the task. The success in achieving any goal is the degree to which it can be measured, as what gets measured is far more likely to be done. The simple task of writing things down greatly increases the likelihood of putting in place the actions that lead toward the dream, and ultimately the likelihood of achieving these dreams. Additionally, writing helps bring order to the mind, which is essential in both building psychological and emotional capacity and allowing effective regeneration in these domains (refer to Chapter 8). The act of writing gives the mind a disciplined means of expression and provides the stimulus to enable the athlete to analyze and understand experiences that are the key to self-awareness (refer to Chapter 5).

The Process

In terms of identifying the dream and taking action to achieve it, the Performance Lifestyle identifies four key elements of the goal-setting process. These steps work together to optimize the effectiveness of this process:

- Identifying the dream
- Identifying the route and markers along the way to the dreams
- Taking action by developing positive rituals
- Reviewing and taking action again

At all times within the Performance Lifestyle, the need to address psychological and emotional fitness along with physical fitness is emphasized. An athlete with a well-balanced life is far more likely to achieve optimal emotional and psychological health, and is therefore likely to optimize recovery and subsequent performance. For this reason, the dream-setting activity should not be restricted to athletics, but should also be carried out for life away from athletics.

For each area, the process will involve writing down the big dream, identifying and writing down any markers along the way to the dream, and tracking daily actions toward the dream. It will then involve monitoring the progress on a regular basis and rebuilding the path toward the goals however and whenever necessary.

Identifying the Dream

A coach should ask his athletes: "In a perfect world with no barriers, what would you like to achieve in life and athletics?" This question is the first and most important question the athlete must address, as the answer is his dream. It is important that the dream is *big*, and each athlete should be encouraged to express what he really wants to achieve, not what someone else wants him to achieve. The size and personalization of the dream is crucial, as only if it is his own dream will he have the required levels of discipline and motivation to fully commit to the achievement of this dream. A positive dream has the power to motivate the athlete to undertake some of the key activities and/or lifestyle changes that will enhance his likelihood of achieving it. A positive approach is vital (refer to Chapter 6). The dream needs to be big enough to ensure that athletes stay in a positive, energized mode whenever they are working toward the dream.

Whatever the dream, it is important that the dream is identified and written down. Ideally, it should be written in a place where the athlete will look at it on a regular basis, as doing so provides positive reinforcement toward undertaking the activities that lead to this dream. Writing it down it makes the dream real and increases the likelihood of achieving it. Figure 4-1 outlines an appropriate dream-setting template.

The Dream

What would you like to achieve in athletics?

How will you know when you have achieved it (what will you see, feel, hear, etc.)?

What are the key milestones you will need to achieve along the way and when would you like to achieve them?

Goals **Dates**

What are the key goals you want to achieve this year?

Goals **Dates**

Figure 4-1

To maximize commitment to the dream, it is important to make this dream pervasive. The more real it appears, the greater its ability to motivate and the greater the likelihood that it will be achieved. An important psychological tool in creating realism is visualization, which needs to be used to make the goal as real as possible. Visualization involves the creation of images in the mind, images that show athletes successfully completing tasks and achieving dreams. Visualization is as effective as the quality of the image developed. Images can be imagined as movies, and the more developed these movies, the more effective they will be in achieving their aims. Movies are at their most effective when all senses are used. Therefore, during visualization sessions, attention needs to be focused not only on the image, but also on the sounds, smells, feelings, and tastes associated with the image. As quality in each of these areas is developed, the quality of the movie is enhanced and the realism associated with the dream is simultaneously enhanced. Figure 4-2 outlines how effective movies can be developed in the mind. These movies can be used in the dream-setting exercise and are also useful in other pillars of the Performance Lifestyle.

Make the Dream a Movie

When you have written down your dream, complete the following activity:

Picture yourself attaining your big dream.

Look at the picture and imagine yourself in the middle of the movie, just as if you are watching yourself achieving your success. Pay attention to the size of the image. Make it as big as possible. Next, look at the colors, making them as vivid as possible. Next, switch up the brightness, just as you would on a TV set. The aim is to make the picture as clear and vivid as possible. Watch this movie for a while.

Next, turn to the sound. Again, play with the controls and make the sounds as loud and real as you can.

Then turn to any smells, tastes, or feelings that you can imagine. This step may be a bit tougher, but remember that the more real the image the better.

This is the image of success. You need to store it and use it at regular intervals. It will help remind you of why you are carrying out all of your actions. Whenever you feel the need for focus and motivation, play this movie in your mind, which will reinforce the reason why you are undertaking that activity.

Figure 4-2

Identifying the Route and Markers Along the Way to the Dreams

In many cases, the ultimate dream will be some way down the road, such as getting a college scholarship or competing in the Olympics. These big dreams are important, but as they are further away, the possibility of being sidetracked is always possible. It is important that the athlete stays on the track toward the dream and remains motivated to undertake the key actions toward this dream. Regular success can provide the impetus to do just that. Success is a great motivator, and by breaking the dream down into small goals, a series of successes can be set up.

Successful completion of tasks can provide the motivation to continue action toward a big dream. To this end, the development of route markers is an important element of maintaining motivation and action, as well as providing a clear direction toward the dream. Anyone setting out on a journey will study a map and draw up a roadmap toward the destination. Similarly, breaking a big dream up into smaller parts, which together build toward the big dream, is a vital aspect of achieving the big dream itself. Once the dream has been identified, it is important that a route is built to move the athlete toward it. While the dream provides the overall direction, it is also important to note markers along the pathway. Just as a roadmap identifies key landmarks to help drivers navigate toward a destination, such markers provide indicators to ensure that athletes are headed in the right direction toward their dreams.

These markers need to be short-term (monthly) and long-term (half-yearly or yearly) to provide for a clear route toward the dream. They can include various measures, such as fitness scores, performance scores, or selection for teams. Figure 4-3 presents a completed dream-setting template and identifies a number of key markers toward the dream.

Once set up, this roadmap will guide the athlete's work program for a given period. It will provide clear targets that need to be achieved, targets that will have been carefully selected to contribute to the achievement of the dream. This route will guide activities and actions undertaken within a given timeframe. Therefore, at any time an athlete should know whether he is on track to achieving his dreams, and what actions he needs to take to ensure he remains on track.

Taking Action by Developing Positive Rituals

Once the roadmap has been identified, the athlete must ensure that he identifies appropriate goals for each month, and these goals must be based on the roadmap. This process needs to be logged in a written account, as doing so adds a level of commitment (Figure 4-4). Each month, the athlete will write down key actions that will move him toward his goal. These actions can then be broken into a small number of weekly goals. The weekly log that is used as a key aspect of Pillar 2 has a section that

The Dream

What would you like to achieve in athletics?

How will you know when you have achieved it (what will you see, feel, hear, etc.)?

I will be leaving the dressing room to the distant roaring sound of the crowd. As I near the arena, the noise will become deafening and the music will be playing on the PA. As I enter the tunnel, a bright light will shine and I will smell the grass. My name will be announced as a starter and I will run out to the sounds of the crowd and the sight of thousands of people wearing the team's colors.

What are the key milestones you will need to achieve along the way, and when would you like to achieve them?

Goals	**Dates**
To start on my high school team	Sophomore year
To run the 40-yard dash in 4.7 seconds	Sophomore year
To run the 40-yard dash in 4.6 seconds	Junior year
To receive interest letters	Junior year
To be selected as an All-State player	Senior year
To gain 30 pounds of lean muscle mass	Senior year
To squat 500 pounds	Senior Year
To run the 40-yard dash in 4.5 seconds	Senior year

What are the key goals you want to achieve this year?

Goals	**Dates**
To gain 10 pounds of lean muscle mass	June
To develop my movement patterns	June
To add 50 pounds to my best squat performance	June
To perfect my clean	June
To run the 40-yard dash in 4.8 seconds	June

Figure 4-3

requires the athlete to identify his key goals for each week, and also an area that asks whether he has taken action toward this goal each day (refer to Chapter 5). This process has two important benefits:

- It reminds the athlete of the need to take action toward his goals.
- It enables the athlete to achieve a positive relaxed state (refer to Chapter 7), knowing that he has undertaken activities toward his goals.

Choosing Words Carefully

The wording of the goals is vital and can have a very large psychological effect on the athlete's subconscious. Effective wording can greatly enhance adherence to the goals,

Monthly Goal Setting

What are your goals for this month?

Week 1: What actions will you take this week to achieve the goals?

Week 2: What actions will you take this week to achieve the goals?

Week 3: What actions will you take this week to achieve the goals?

Week 4: What actions will you take this week to achieve the goals?

Figure 4-4

while ineffective wording can greatly increase the likelihood of failure. Effective goals should follow the following three key guidelines for effective goals, as outlined by Michael Heppell in his book *How to Be Brilliant*. To maximize effectiveness, the wording of goals needs to be:

- Personal: All goals must be personal to the athlete. They must always be framed with the word "I." For example "I eat breakfast each morning." This wording ensures that the responsibility for taking the action lies with the person. Similarly, the benefits associated with the action will accrue directly to the individual.
- Positive: All goals must be worded positively. This wording implies movement toward a goal, rather than away from an action. A goal of improving nutrition should be worded as, "I eat three pieces of fruit a day" (a positive action), rather than "I will avoid eating chocolate," which is negatively worded. The emphasis of the former is on the healthy action, while the latter goal focuses on the unhealthy action. Additionally, the first wording implies action. It is important to avoid weak words, such as "try," which implies that the task will be difficult. Imagine a goal worded as, "I will try to get to bed by 10:00 each night." This goal is simply set up to fail. If this goal is reworded as, "I get to bed by 10:00 each night," and written down and shared with someone else, then the goal is far more likely to be achieved.
- Present: All goals should be worded in the present. This technique is another key empowerment method, as present-tense goals imply that the goal has been achieved, and the mind supposes this situation to be true. Again, the phrase used earlier, "I eat three pieces of fruit per day," is worded in the present to imply that the action is already being achieved, which helps the mind turn the goal into reality.

As with all aspects of this pillar, the athlete must commit to writing the goals down and logging any action taken. These goals need to be written in a place where they can be seen, rather than being locked away, as visibility reinforces their effectiveness. Again, the training/recovery log provides an ideal medium, as this document is viewed and worked on daily.

Additionally, sharing the goal with another person can motivate the athlete to achieve it. For example, if another person knows that the athlete's goal is to be in bed by 10:00, then that person can reinforce this goal at times when it is not being achieved. Clearly, the choice of person to share with may vary with the goal, and this sharing implies a level of trust between the athlete and the other person.

Vision Without Action is a Daydream

At this point, the athlete will have a dream, a route to the dream, and key actions and goals for a given time period. Unfortunately, this point is where many goal-setting programs fall down, as the next part—taking action—is crucial to whether or not the dream will become a reality. Unless athletes actually do something about achieving their dreams, chances are they will remain nothing more than daydreams. While dreams and goals are all well and good, they are useless unless positive action is taken to achieve them.

A key method by which goals will be achieved and actions will be taken within the Performance Lifestyle is through the efficacious use of rituals. The importance of rituals is fully discussed in Chapter 7, but it is important that they are examined in this context as well, as they play an important role in achieving goals. Rituals are actions taken without the need for a great deal of thought, and thus are low in energy demand.

Many of the key goals that an athlete will identify will be achievable through rituals. Actions such as always eating breakfast, going to bed earlier, and always cooling down after sessions are best developed as rituals. While these behaviors would need to be listed as goal activities in the early stages of this process, once they have become rituals they would not need to be listed in weekly goals, unless the ritual breaks down at some point. Developing a few rituals at a time enables the athlete to subconsciously make a number of key daily decisions that can really increase his recovery capacity.

Reviewing and Taking Action Again

At the end of each month, athletes need to review their progress. They need to analyze which goals were achieved, which goals were not, and the factors that contributed to the success or failure. Factors that contribute to success would be reinforced, while factors that contribute to failure may become the basis for the next month's goals. For example, a goal of getting to bed by 10:00 might have been compromised by the need to complete schoolwork. A new goal of setting aside an hour for schoolwork during the day would then become key. Success in this capacity would allow for effective schoolwork and would also lead to the ability to get to bed at an earlier time.

Figure 4-5 shows how goals can be reviewed, allows an athlete to look at how successful he was in achieving his goals, and identifies reasons why he was or was not able to achieve them. Using this information, he can then plan out the next month of work. This process needs to become a monthly ritual, whereby the athlete takes stock of progress and then plans the next month's actions. Figure 4-6 shows a completed monthly review.

Just as progress toward any task needs to be monitored, monitoring progress toward the dream is essential, and the route-markers provide appropriate ways in which to monitor progress. However, it must be remembered that lives, both within and outside athletics, change rapidly. It is important, therefore, to view the markers simply as guidelines and not as set in stone. They need to be regularly evaluated and

Monthly Goal Analysis

What were your goals for this month?

How successful were you in achieving these goals?

What factors helped you achieve the goals?

What factors hindered you in achieving the goals?

Figure 4-5

Monthly Goal Analysis

What were your goals for this month?

To eat breakfast each day
To get eight hours of sleep per night
To look at poor performances with a positive perspective

How successful were you in achieving these goals?

I was able to get eight hours of sleep per night by going to bed each night at 10:00 pm. Once this routine was set, I found it quite easy to make sure I got the sleep. This extra sleep helped my performances, as I felt I had a lot more energy. By feeling fresher in the morning, I was able to have time for breakfast, which in turn helped my energy levels.

While my performances were generally better, at times when they were not as good as I would like. I still blamed myself and questioned my ability, which I found sapped my energy levels.

What factors helped you achieve the goals?

Establishing a regular routine really helped.
Seeing the effects of the changes helped me realize the need for them.

What factors hindered you in achieving the goals?

I am still critical of my performances and dwell on them.

Figure 4-6

reset. Injuries, for example, may make the attainment of some performance goals unrealistic. In this case, it is important that the athlete takes stock of progress to date and then sets new markers that relate to the given situation (e.g., to rebuild fitness levels to their pre-injury levels by a given date).

Identifying and Addressing the Basic Individual Needs

It is most likely that the dream-setting experience to date has involved athletic goals. However, in terms of recovery, it is important that an athlete meets all of his basic needs as well as those in athletics. Achieving an effective life balance, together with emotional, physical, and psychological fitness, is a key aspect of the Performance Lifestyle. All people, of all ages, will have basic underlying human needs. Again, these needs may be related to athletics, but they will often involve aspects away from athletics of which the athlete and his coach should be aware. While the primary dream is often clear, these needs are more difficult to ascertain at first and may come at a subconscious or secondary level.

The first step in identifying these needs is to get the athlete to sit down quietly and write down things that make him feel good. These things should bring him real pleasure and gratification. Once he has identified these facts, he needs to go further and write down why they bring such pleasure. This secondary investigation will often identify the underlying needs. If he finds this difficult, get him to imagine that he has just returned from the doctor, who told him that he only has one more week to live. Given this timeframe, what would he do? This scenario will often help athletes identify what they value most. Figure 4-7 provides a template by which this process can be carried out.

Facts that arise may include time spent with family or loved ones, time to spend on an interest or hobby, or time spent with friends. Again, this process will likely involve issues related to athletics, but also issues away from the athletic arena. While the athletic issues are normally easy to achieve (e.g., time spent with teammates, the big match atmosphere), all too often the other needs are overlooked in the quest for athletic glory. However, any need not met creates a potential energy drain. While this energy drain often is not evident in reduced performance in the short term, if it is not addressed the long-term consequences can have large repercussions on performance, as illustrated by the case study presented in Figure 4-8.

My Real Values

If you were going to die in a week, what would you do with this time?

After you've gone, how would you like to be remembered?

What activities give you the most satisfaction?

Why do you feel these activities give you satisfaction?

What do you think your major life needs are, and how well are you addressing them at present?

Figure 4-7

Case Study

A committed college athlete spends a massive deal of time enhancing his athletic performance with activities such as practice time, studying plays, strength and conditioning, etc. Additionally, he has to keep up with schoolwork, etc. Given this massive time commitment, he simply did not have time to be able to engage in his hobby of playing the guitar, which brought him a great deal of pleasure in high school and which was a great relaxation activity. In the short term, this absence did not have a large effect, but as time went on the athlete came to resent the extra video sessions, lifting sessions, etc., and yearned for some time to spend playing the guitar. This situation resulted in feelings of anger and resentment toward the game and the coaches. Increasingly, this athlete found himself reluctantly going through training rather then loving the training. As training became a chore, his performance level, rather then improving, started to plateau and then decline. The coach then required extra work, leaving even less free time for the athlete. Eventually, the athlete became disheartened and quit.

In this scenario, had the athlete identified the true importance of his hobby, he could have initiated a positive ritual to ensure that he devoted some time to the guitar each week. Had this change occurred, then his frustration with the time commitments would have been greatly reduced and the anger and frustration would not have been evident. Thus, the energy drain would have been removed and his performance would have continued to improve.

Figure 4-8

Developing Positive Lifestyle Rituals

Positive rituals, as discussed earlier, are a pillar of the Performance Lifestyle (refer to Chapter 7), and have already been identified as a key to achieving any dream. Additionally, rituals are fundamental to ensuring that the athlete is able to commit time to his own life needs. Once these main needs are identified, it is important that rituals are put in place to ensure that the athlete is able to meet these needs. As an example, the athlete described in Figure 4-8 could devote one hour per week to playing the guitar. This time would be set and the athlete would then stick to this ritual on a weekly basis. Doing so would ensure that this time is always devoted to one of his key identified needs. Figure 4-9 provides a template for setting up rituals to address an athlete's life needs, while Figure 4-10 shows a completed template.

My Life Needs

What things in life are most important to you?

How successful are you at ensuring that these needs are met?

How will you make sure that you address these needs (the rituals you will follow)?

Figure 4-9

My Life Needs

What things in life are most important to you?

My family is the most important thing in my life.

Becoming the best baseball player I can be

Financial security

Using my strengths as a student

How successful are you at ensuring that these needs are met?

With my training regimen at present, I am not spending enough time with my family.

I am attending to my athletic development well, and feel my performance improvements are excellent.

With the emphasis on athletics, I am not able to devote as much time to my studies, and am unable to utilize my learning abilities. This situation might affect my financial security. If I fail to make it in baseball, I may not have anything to fall back on.

How will you make sure that you address these needs (the rituals you will follow)?

I will spend two hours each Sunday visiting and spending quality time with my family.

I will call my family each Wednesday and devote at least a half hour to talking about them, rather than about me.

I will spend an hour each day on my studies, rather than playing on computer games. This action will help maintain my love of learning and also ensure I have a fall-back option in terms of my financial security.

Figure 4-10

Summary

- Clear goals, together with feedback, are a vital part of achieving optimal functioning.
- With clear goals and feedback, psychic energy is invested in activities that move an athlete forward.
- The athlete needs to have a clear dream, as well as route-markers toward this dream. These dreams and route-markers need to be written down and kept where they are regularly in view.
- Taking action is vital to achieving goals and involves setting clear actions on a monthly and weekly basis and then reviewing them regularly.
- Rituals are the key to effective actions.
- Goals need to involve life needs as well as athletic goals.

5

Pillar 2— Developing Self-Awareness

"Know thyself."
—Written on the Oracle at Delphi

How do athletes know when they are experiencing underrecovery? This question is key in the quest to proactively dealing with the problems associated with this condition. Stress and fatigue, by their multidimensional nature, will manifest in very different ways within a group of individuals. Therefore, it is unlikely that a single sign will indicate underrecovery in all athletes, as proven by the range of symptoms associated with this phenomenon. Given this unique individual nature of fatigue and recovery, an individualized approach to optimizing recovery is essential. This situation can present a great challenge for any coach, as individualizing an approach for every athlete can be enormously time-consuming. The most effective way of achieving this objective is to empower the athletes to become aware of their unique sources of stress, together with their typical responses to these stressors. Athletes are then able to identify sources of stress within their lives and anticipate times when these stressors will appear. Additionally, they are empowered to make appropriate lifestyle decisions that enhance recovery and performance, and make appropriate interventions whenever additional stress occurs.

This empowerment is the basis of the Performance Lifestyle, and self-awareness is fundamental to achieving an individualized recovery program. While educating athletes in the methods of recovery is a vital part of "empowerment," an equally important element is for the athletes to become aware of their levels of recovery and performance in all domains. Athletes need to be constantly asking themselves key performance questions, such as the following:

- Am I enjoying my training?
- What are my energy levels like?
- What is my performance like?
- Do I feel recovered?

These questions develop an athlete's self-awareness of his recovery levels. This pillar develops a structured method by which this awareness can be developed.

Because fitness is multidimensional, it is essential that self-awareness is developed in all domains—physical, psychological, and emotional. An athlete can become aware of his levels of stress and subsequent recovery in all three domains, and then make appropriate adaptations to deal with the specific stressors.

Self-Monitoring for Self-Awareness

A key to developing the essential skill of self-awareness is utilizing self-monitoring. By using this tool, the potential for developing self-awareness is greatly enhanced. Just as for Pillar 1, actively monitoring via a formal written assessment greatly enhances the effectiveness of the self-monitoring process. Attention is drawn to key factors relating to recovery. This process develops a heightened level of self-awareness, which then helps the athlete put in place any changes required to enhance recovery. This self-monitoring will involve identifying levels and sources of stress, levels of recovery, and the effects of different recovery techniques. This process provides a level of control, which in itself can enhance the recovery process, with each athlete empowered to take individualized actions to deal with his unique situation. Self-monitoring is an important aspect of the education of any athlete and fundamental to the development of the empowered athlete, which lies at the heart of the Performance Lifestyle.

Areas for Awareness Development

Because fitness and recovery occur in three domains, it makes sense that awareness needs to be developed in all three domains as well. The Performance Lifestyle has developed systems that relate to performance in all domains. Therefore, the self-awareness pillar has three main processes that encompass the three domains of fitness.

- Monitoring athletic performance and recovery
- Lifestyle and emotional monitoring
- Psychological profiling

A key in any process is compliance. The systems outlined in this chapter can provide very powerful information, but do not take an inordinate amount of time to complete. Integrating the performance- and recovery-monitoring system with the training log allows athletes to evaluate both training stress and subsequent recovery with the same tool.

While more sophisticated techniques exist that measure awareness more fully in different domains, these techniques are often time-consuming and are not always feasible for many athletes. Athletes are encouraged to use these tools if they feel the need to investigate certain domains of recovery in more depth.

Monitoring Performance and Recovery

The aim of the performance self-monitoring process is to enable athletes to develop the knowledge and skills to help them identify their levels of physical performance and identify their levels of recovery. If this process is effective, an athlete will become aware of times when recovery is less than optimal, and of the need to be proactive to enhance recovery at these times.

To evaluate the level of an athlete's performance and recovery, the training/recovery log system has been developed that allows the athlete to combine data related to performance levels, training loads, and levels of recovery. Taken together, this information provides a powerful tool for both physical self-awareness and physical-performance analysis. This tool gives an athlete a good picture of his levels of athletic performance and recovery.

The Training/Recovery Log

Optimal performance, as explained earlier, is intricately linked to training and subsequent recovery. Because training and recovery are so closely linked, it is pertinent to combine the data from the training log with key indicators of recovery. In addition, an area is set aside for general comments on factors related to non-training stress and emotional states, as these issues are also closely linked to optimal performance. The system also includes information about weekly goals, daily goal activity, and nutrition quality, and provides a powerful source of information for the athlete (Figure 5-1).

Using the System

In the beginning of the recording sheet, athletes are required to identify the training week, training phase (e.g., preparatory, precompetition), and their weekly goals, as identified in Pillar 1. This step is important, as it helps reinforce the work they are carrying out to reach their stated goals.

Identifying the training periods also helps reinforce the aims of each training phase. For example, it can help identify periods of planned over-reaching that are included in

TRAINING AND RECOVERY LOG

Date: ______________________ Phase of Training ______________________

This week's goals: ____

____

____

MON	RECOVERY		OTHER TRAINING	TEAM PRACTICE
Wake Wt [ ] Wake HR [ ] Hrs sleep [ ]	General health Appetite Motivation Energy levels Muscle soreness Sleep quality Work quality	5 4 3 2 1 5 4 3 2 1 5 4 3 2 1 5 4 3 2 1 5 4 3 2 1 5 4 3 2 1 5 4 3 2 1	Time___ Dur ___ RPE___	Time___ Dur ___ RPE___

LIFTING SESSION Time				
Exercise	Wt/R	Wt/R	Wt/R	Wt/R

GENERAL COMMENTS	
Recovery techniques used	
Goal action taken Yes No	
General nutrition 5 4 3 2 1	Perf score

TUES	RECOVERY		OTHER TRAINING	TEAM PRACTICE
Wake Wt [ ] Wake HR [ ] Hrs sleep [ ]	General health Appetite Motivation Energy levels Muscle soreness Sleep quality Work quality	5 4 3 2 1 5 4 3 2 1 5 4 3 2 1 5 4 3 2 1 5 4 3 2 1 5 4 3 2 1 5 4 3 2 1	Time___ Dur ___ RPE___	Time___ Dur ___ RPE___

LIFTING SESSION Time				
Exercise	Wt/R	Wt/R	Wt/R	Wt/R

GENERAL COMMENTS	
Recovery techniques used	
Goal action taken Yes No	
General nutrition 5 4 3 2 1	Perf score

Figure 5-1

WED	RECOVERY		OTHER TRAINING	TEAM PRACTICE
Wake Wt Wake HR Hrs sleep	General health Appetite Motivation Energy levels Muscle soreness Sleep quality Work quality	5 4 3 2 1 5 4 3 2 1 5 4 3 2 1 5 4 3 2 1 5 4 3 2 1 5 4 3 2 1 5 4 3 2 1	Time___ Dur ___ RPE___	Time___ Dur ___ RPE___

LIFTING SESSION Time

Exercise	Wt/R	Wt/R	Wt/R	Wt/R

GENERAL COMMENTS

Recovery techniques used

Goal action taken Yes No

General nutrition 5 4 3 2 1 | Perf score

THURS	RECOVERY		OTHER TRAINING	TEAM PRACTICE
Wake Wt Wake HR Hrs sleep	General health Appetite Motivation Energy levels Muscle soreness Sleep quality Work quality	5 4 3 2 1 5 4 3 2 1 5 4 3 2 1 5 4 3 2 1 5 4 3 2 1 5 4 3 2 1 5 4 3 2 1	Time___ Dur ___ RPE___	Time___ Dur ___ RPE___

LIFTING SESSION Time

Exercise	Wt/R	Wt/R	Wt/R	Wt/R

GENERAL COMMENTS

Recovery techniques used

Goal action taken Yes No

General nutrition 5 4 3 2 1 | Perf score

FRI	RECOVERY		OTHER TRAINING	TEAM PRACTICE
Wake Wt Wake HR Hrs sleep	General health Appetite Motivation Energy levels Muscle soreness Sleep quality Work quality	5 4 3 2 1 5 4 3 2 1 5 4 3 2 1 5 4 3 2 1 5 4 3 2 1 5 4 3 2 1 5 4 3 2 1	Time___ Dur ___ RPE___	Time___ Dur ___ RPE___

LIFTING SESSION Time

Exercise	Wt/R	Wt/R	Wt/R	Wt/R

GENERAL COMMENTS

Recovery techniques used

Goal action taken Yes No

General nutrition 5 4 3 2 1 | Perf score

Figure 5-1 cont

SAT	RECOVERY		OTHER TRAINING	TEAM PRACTICE
Wake Wt Wake HR Hrs sleep	General health Appetite Motivation Energy levels Muscle soreness Sleep quality Work quality	5 4 3 2 1 5 4 3 2 1 5 4 3 2 1 5 4 3 2 1 5 4 3 2 1 5 4 3 2 1 5 4 3 2 1	Time___ Dur ___ RPE___	Time___ Dur ___ RPE___

LIFTING SESSION Time					GENERAL COMMENTS	
Exercise	Wt/R	Wt/R	Wt/R	Wt/R		
					Recovery techniques used	
					Goal action taken Yes No	
					General nutrition 5 4 3 2 1	Perf score

SUN	RECOVERY		OTHER TRAINING	TEAM PRACTICE
Wake Wt Wake HR Hrs sleep	General health Appetite Motivation Energy levels Muscle soreness Sleep quality Work quality	5 4 3 2 1 5 4 3 2 1 5 4 3 2 1 5 4 3 2 1 5 4 3 2 1 5 4 3 2 1 5 4 3 2 1	Time___ Dur ___ RPE___	Time___ Dur ___ RPE___

LIFTING SESSION Time					GENERAL COMMENTS	
Exercise	Wt/R	Wt/R	Wt/R	Wt/R		
					Recovery techniques used	
					Goal action taken Yes No	
					General nutrition 5 4 3 2 1	Perf score

Figure 5-1 cont

the program, where deterioration in the quality of scores is expected. This process helps an athlete appropriately relate his performance feedback, and reinforces the fact that performance peaks cannot be maintained throughout the year. However, even during periods of planned overreaching, the form helps identify whether the athlete can tolerate high levels of overreaching-type training without having excessive symptoms of underrecovery, and helps provide appropriate training loads.

The athlete then rates his level of nonathletic stress. Remember, stress tolerance can break down from a sudden increase in overall stress, not just from an increase in physical distress. This type of stress needs to be accounted for when setting the training programs, and allows coaches and athletes to respond to periods when athletes may be under excessive stress, such as exam periods. The programs should also include the stress caused by the emotional demands of competition. This process helps emphasize the inter-relationship between lifestyle and performance.

The rest of the form then consists of daily recording of key data and training information that relates to physiological, psychological, and emotional symptoms of underrecovery. Athletes are asked to record a number of key parameters, both objective and subjective, that contribute to the picture the coach and athletes will get of how the athletes are responding to the training stimuli being set, and how they are recovering from each session.

The key objective measures are the resting heart rate and waking body weight. The number of hours of sleep is also recorded, as sleep is an important factor for all athletes. Inadequate sleep can, by itself, be a cause of underrecovery. Either the resting heart rate rising or the body weight falling for a period of three days could be an early indicator of underrecovery.

The athlete then takes a subjective measure of sleep quality via a 5-point Likert scale. This 5-point scale is used for all of the subjective measures. On the scale, 5 represents a great score and 1 represents a poor score. While inter-athlete variation may exist when using the scale (i.e., one athlete's 5 may be another athlete's 4), what is more important is the consistency within each athlete.

The form then serves as a normal training log. During the day, the athlete records his training or competition for that day. It is important that the athlete records all physical activities, including running sessions, team practices, and any physical recreation he undertakes. Doing so allows the total physical load to be evaluated, as opposed to just the load from strength-training sessions, for example. Logging strength sessions involves recording the exercises, sets, reps, and resistances used.

All other training activities should be logged, including the activities undertaken, and the time, duration, and intensity of the sessions. Energy expenditure is affected by both training volume (how long a person trains) and training intensity (how hard a person trains). Taken together, these factors will affect the overall level of energy expenditure and the overall level of stress. The intensity of the session can be recorded using a session exertion rating, which is a modified ratings of perceived exertion scale (Figure 5-2). The athletes should also record whether they used recovery techniques during that day, as doing so contributes to the capacity to recover and further emphasizes the proactive approach to recovery they need to take.

Session Exertion Rating	
Rating	
0	Nothing
1	Extremely light
2	Very light
3	Light
4	Light to moderate
5	Moderate
6	Moderate to hard
7	Hard
8	Very hard
9	Extremely hard
10	Maximal effort

Figure 5-2

The athlete then makes five subjective measures of factors relating to underrecovery, all selected to reflect physical, psychological, and emotional measures. An athlete records his score for general health, appetite, motivation to train, general energy levels, performance level, and level of muscle soreness—all factors identified as symptoms of overtraining. Taken together, these factors provide a very powerful, multidimensional insight into overall recovery. Wherever scores drop, especially if they reach 2 or below, they can be early indicators of underrecovery and can be the trigger to initiate additional recovery or stress-reducing activities.

This identification process can be supplemented by the use of performance scores where appropriate. Whenever an athlete undertakes a fitness test with a high neural requirement (such as speed, agility, and power scores), the result can be recorded (e.g., 10-yard dash in 1.63 seconds). These tests do not need to be sought out (i.e., they do not have to be regular activities) and should only be used when they occur during normal activities. However, when they are used, they should be incorporated into the log, as they provide powerful performance-evaluation tools. Reduced performance in these neural-dependent activities can be an early indicator of underrecovery.

General Comments

This area should be seen as both a training diary and a general diary on thoughts feelings, emotions, etc. The athlete should record everything that pertains to both his performance and his quality of life. This process can include commenting on any of the facts highlighted within the recording, such as energy levels, performance levels, etc., but should also include anything the athlete feels is impacting his life and performance. The key to developing psychological and emotional capacities is to become aware of these emotions. This section should be used to record thoughts and feelings. By writing these things down, the athlete acknowledges them and can identify patterns of how and when they occur. It is also key to building the required capacity in these domains. At the same time, the athlete needs to go deeper than the emotion itself, and ask himself why he is feeling a certain way, as doing so will assist in developing the positive outlook covered in Chapter 6. As the athlete's emotional intelligence increases, this area will increasingly include more diverse areas that may not have previously been seen as related to performance. This area should never be limited; instead, the athlete should be encouraged to write as freely as possible. The act of writing is, in itself, a great release. Writing down problems can often make the problems look trivial and greatly reduce their energy-sapping capacity. This section of the log is a great disengagement strategy (refer to Chapter 8), and is closely linked to the "power of positive" (refer to Chapter 6). Figure 5-3 provides an example of a completed daily log.

MON		RECOVERY		OTHER TRAINING	TEAM PRACTICE
Wake Wt	196	General health	5 **4** 3 2 1	Time___ Dur___ RPE___	Time 2:00; Dur 2 hours; RPE 6
Wake HR	64	Appetite	5 4 **3** 2 1		Noncontact team practice, ran through all plays for the game. Not too strenuous, but a large number of high-quality runs.
Hrs sleep	6	Motivation	5 4 **3** 2 1		
		Energy levels	5 4 **3** 2 1		
		Muscle soreness	5 4 3 **2** 1		
		Sleep quality	5 4 3 **2** 1		
		Work quality	5 4 **3** 2 1		

LIFTING SESSION	Time			
Exercise	Wt/R	Wt/R	Wt/R	Wt/R
Cleans	220/3	230/3	230/3	230/3
Jerk	180/4	190/3	200/3	
Squats	300/8	320/6	330/5	340/4
Romanian dead lift	240/6	250/6	250/6	

GENERAL COMMENTS

Felt a little jaded today, although my weights were okay, my power output seemed down. Also, I didn't feel sharp in the team practice. Felt a little sore this morning and didn't sleep so well last night, waking a number of times. Used the ice bath after training and got a massage. The exams are starting to cause me anxiety. I need to get a lot of work done, but can't fit it in. Also, I'm having some trouble with my girlfriend because she wants me to spend more time with her, but I just haven't got the time.

Recovery techniques used: Ice baths, massage

Goal action taken: Yes ✓ No

General nutrition: 5 4 **3** 2 1 | Performance score:

Note: Wt/R = Weight/repetitions

Figure 5-3

The initial signs of underrecovery are evident in Figure 5-3. Performance is less than optimal, especially in relation to the neural-dominant aspects such as speed and power, which are often the first aspects to deteriorate. Additionally, some of the key indicators of underrecovery are scoring at 3 or less. In response to this situation, the athlete has undertaken some proactive recovery activities.

The general comments section identifies some possible causes of additional stress, which will need to be addressed. Examination stress, along with the stress of the athlete's relationship, is likely contributing to this underrecovered state.

The log has identified the earl signs of underrecovery, allowing the athlete to take action before the situation becomes too serious. It has also identified some possible causes of this underrecovery in areas that may not initially be obvious, and that a coach would be unlikely to pick up.

Lifestyle and Emotional Monitoring

How is an athlete's lifestyle contributing to energy levels and subsequent recovery ability? This question is key in any recovery program. The lifestyle profile can help an athlete assess areas of his lifestyle that are contributing energy and those that are potential energy sappers. Information gained from these areas closely relates to the performance quadrant, which is discussed in Chapter 6. In that pillar, the importance of staying in the positive parts of the quadrant is outlined. However, it is important to realize that everybody, at some time, will enter the negative half. This moment is inevitable and needs to happen to fully develop a person's capacities. It will happen both during activity (i.e., games or practice) and during a person's everyday life.

The principles of the Performance Lifestyle state that stressors are additive and can occur from all domains of fitness. Thus, an awareness of the source of stressors is an important element of self-awareness. The following components of lifestyle are common sources of non-training-related stressors.

Sleep

Sleep is vital for full recovery. Therefore, a problem with either sleep quality or quantity can have a significant effect on performance. It is important that an athlete identifies sleep problems as early as possible and explores methods of dealing with any problems. This issue is discussed further in Chapter 10, and the lifestyle profile allows potential problems to be identified.

Nutrition

Nutrition can have an important effect on the ability to recover from workouts, not to mention overall health. The role of nutrition is covered fully in Chapter 9, but again the lifestyle profile allows potential problems to be identified.

Life Management

At all times, it is important to remember that athletes have a life away from athletics that provides the potential for both energizing and energy-sapping activities to take place. The athlete needs to manage this time effectively in terms of balancing athletic commitments with life commitments, and also managing his lifestyle to provide for an effective Performance Lifestyle. The need for interests and relaxation time away from athletics is important and is stressed within the profile, and the answers give the coach an idea of how an athlete is managing his time and the levels of stress he is bringing to each practice.

Social Relationships

Social relationships have the potential to be uplifting or debilitating. An athlete will be affected by both primary relationships (family) and secondary relationships (schoolmates, team, coaches, etc.). It is important that the athlete can evaluate the effectiveness of his relationships in these areas and identify any areas that are negatively affecting him. Psychologists often stress the importance of strong social support mechanisms in providing the ideal environment for optimum performance, and the feedback can help identify any areas that might be causing the athlete undue stress.

Lifestyle Issues

This area deals with any activities the athlete may be involved in that will compromise performance. Substance abuse, whether it is drugs, alcohol, or tobacco, can have a major debilitating effect on performance, especially when this activity becomes addictive. Similarly, other activities that an athlete may use for excitement or release, such as gambling, have the potential to sap energy and affect recovery levels. Identifying these issues and the level of control an athlete has in his life can assist the athlete in making effective lifestyle decisions. For legal reasons, you may not require the athlete to answer any questions relating to drug abuse, but can include them as a reminder.

The Lifestyle Profile

Figure 5-4 outlines a sample lifestyle profile that can be used to identify areas of non-training-related stress. The scores range from 1 (a poor score) to 10 (a good score). The questions relate to the five main areas of non-training-related stress:

- Sleep patterns (questions 1–5)
- Nutritional patterns (Questions 6–9)
- Life management (Questions 10–19)
- Social relationships, both primary and secondary (Questions 20–24)
- Lifestyle issues (Questions 25–28)

Scores under 5 represent possible problem areas that need to be tackled. The key area identified needs to be highlighted, and strategies and rituals should be put in place to address this issue (refer to Chapter 7). This profile can easily be adapted to relate more effectively to any coach's environment, and questions can be added or removed to increase the relevance to the athletes that you work with.

Psychological Profiling

The way an athlete thinks greatly affects his behavior. Appropriate psychological development is crucial to both effective performance and effective recovery. Chapter 8 reviews the need to both build capacity and recover in the psychological domain. A key aspect of any training program is to target areas that will contribute to increased capacity.

Just as an athlete will use fitness-testing data to evaluate performance and identify areas that need to be developed, the same needs to be done for psychological performance. Figure 5-5 is an adapted version of the competitive adjective profile developed by Jim Loehr (1994). This tool can identify areas of psychological performance that need to be developed. The results of this profile will become the basis of the psychological element of Pillar 4, which is presented in Chapter 7.

Summary

- Self-awareness is essential if athletes are going be able to take effective proactive measures to anticipate or cope with high levels of stress.
- Self-monitoring systems assist the development of self-awareness.
- Self-awareness needs to be developed in all three domains of fitness.
- The recovery/training log is a key tool in the development of self-awareness.
- This process can be supplemented by lifestyle and psychological profiles.

Lifestyle Profile

The Scale

I always get 8 hours sleep per night.	10	9	8	7	6	5	4	3	2	1	I never get 8 hours sleep per night.
My sleep is always of a good quality.	10	9	8	7	6	5	4	3	2	1	My sleep is never of a good quality.
I have a pattern of bed and waking times.	10	9	8	7	6	5	4	3	2	1	I have no pattern of bed and waking times.
I wake naturally each morning.	10	9	8	7	6	5	4	3	2	1	I never wake naturally in the morning.
I wake energized and motivated.	10	9	8	7	6	5	4	3	2	1	I wake listless and unmotivated.
I take in sufficient calories daily.	10	9	8	7	6	5	4	3	2	1	I do not take in sufficient calories daily.
I eat healthily at all times.	10	9	8	7	6	5	4	3	2	1	I never eat healthily.
I always eat breakfast.	10	9	8	7	6	5	4	3	2	1	I never eat breakfast.
I always refuel immediately after exercise.	10	9	8	7	6	5	4	3	2	1	I never refuel immediately after exercise.
I am able to manage my time effectively.	10	9	8	7	6	5	4	3	2	1	I cannot manage my time effectively.
I have no academic worries.	10	9	8	7	6	5	4	3	2	1	I have huge academic worries.
I have no financial worries.	10	9	8	7	6	5	4	3	2	1	I have many financial worries.
My other work schedules are realistic and in balance.	10	9	8	7	6	5	4	3	2	1	My other work schedules are unrealistic and out of balance
I go to bed each night relaxed and unworried.	10	9	8	7	6	5	4	3	2	1	I go to bed each night stressed and worried.
I am able to find at least an hour of rest and relaxation time each day.	10	9	8	7	6	5	4	3	2	1	I am never able to find at least an hour of rest and relaxation time each day.
I have interests and activities that help me relax.	10	9	8	7	6	5	4	3	2	1	I have no interests and activities that help me to relax.
I am in charge of me.	10	9	8	7	6	5	4	3	2	1	I have little control over my life.
Travelling commitments do not sap me of energy.	10	9	8	7	6	5	4	3	2	1	Travelling commitments sap me of energy.

Figure 5-4

Lifestyle Profile

I enjoy my sport.	10	9	8	7	6	5	4	3	2	1	I don't enjoy my sport.
My family life is relaxed and energizing.	10	9	8	7	6	5	4	3	2	1	My family life is stressful and de-energizing
My social relationships are relaxed and energizing.	10	9	8	7	6	5	4	3	2	1	My social relationships are stressful and de-energizing.
My social life never impinges on my performance.	10	9	8	7	6	5	4	3	2	1	My social life always impinges on my performance.
I have great relationships with my teammates.	10	9	8	7	6	5	4	3	2	1	I have poor relationships with my teammates.
I have great relationships with my coaches.	10	9	8	7	6	5	4	3	2	1	I have poor relationships with my coaches.
I never drink alcohol.	10	9	8	7	6	5	4	3	2	1	I drink alcohol on most days.
My alcohol intake when I drink is minimal.	10	9	8	7	6	5	4	3	2	1	My alcohol intake on the days I drink is heavy.
I never smoke.	10	9	8	7	6	5	4	3	2	1	I smoke heavily.
I never take drugs.	10	9	8	7	6	5	4	3	2	1	I take drugs regularly.

Figure 5-4 cont.

Psychological Performance Profile

	The Scale										
I am very competitive.	10	9	8	7	6	5	4	3	2	1	I am not very competitive.
I rely on my own abilities.	10	9	8	7	6	5	4	3	2	1	I rely on other peoples' skills.
I can take control during a game.	10	9	8	7	6	5	4	3	2	1	I rarely take control during a game.
I have confidence in my abilities.	10	9	8	7	6	5	4	3	2	1	I have little confidence in my abilities.
I am able to control my emotions during a game.	10	9	8	7	6	5	4	3	2	1	I am unable to control my emotions during a game.
I am able to bounce back from knocks very quickly.	10	9	8	7	6	5	4	3	2	1	I am unable to bounce back from knocks.
I am disciplined.	10	9	8	7	6	5	4	3	2	1	I am undisciplined.
I am optimistic.	10	9	8	7	6	5	4	3	2	1	I am pessimistic.
I can be flexible in my approach.	10	9	8	7	6	5	4	3	2	1	I am very inflexible in my approach.
I am able to always put out a confident exterior, regardless of how I feel.	10	9	8	7	6	5	4	3	2	1	I am unable to put out a confident exterior when I don't feel confident.
I can focus my attention on getting key tasks done.	10	9	8	7	6	5	4	3	2	1	I am not able to focus my attention on getting key tasks done.
I find tough competition challenging.	10	9	8	7	6	5	4	3	2	1	I am frightened of tough competition.

Figure 5-5

6

Pillar 3—The Power of Positive

"If you are pained by external things, it is not they that disturb you but your own judgment about them."
—Marcus Aurelius

Everyone has met people who are unbelievably positive and seem to energize all situations. Likewise, everyone has met those negative people who seem to sap the energy out of each and every situation. Coaches should teach athletes to look at these people and evaluate their probable levels of physical performance. Invariably, the positive people come out on top. Emotions, beliefs, and thoughts play a vital role in the body's functions and have the capacity to either enhance or retard recovery. What makes this concept especially important is that every athlete is able to shape his own memories, thoughts, and feelings, and then create himself through the way in which he invests his energy.

This pillar demonstrates how being positive can greatly enhance the likelihood of achieving successful performance and recovery, and is fundamental to long-term energy capacity and recovery. While being positive cannot guarantee successful recovery and performance, negativity will certainly guarantee less than optimal recovery and performance. Creating a positive mindset is vital to recovery and the key is the effective use of energy. Whenever an athlete needs to build capacity, it is important that he channels his energy into productive activities. Similarly, when an athlete recovers, it is important that he minimizes energy leaks, conserves energy, and maximizes recovery. To do so, the athlete must become aware of the ideal Performance Lifestyle mood state. Mihaly Csikszentmihalyi (2002) describes this optimal mood state as flow, or "a state of joy, creativity, and total involvement in which problems seem to disappear and where there is an exhilarating feeling of transcendence." This flow mood state presents an optimal model for both performance and recovery, with the only difference being the levels of energy being expended in each situation.

The Ideal Performance Lifestyle Mood State

All moods and thoughts can be placed on a continuum between positive and negative. Additionally, they can be placed on a continuum between high energy and low energy. Anger, for example, is a high-energy emotion, but it is also a negative emotion. Anger has the potential to significantly sap energy, especially when it persists for an extended time. Enthusiasm, on the other hand, is a high-energy but positive emotion that creates an energized situation. Contentment is a low-energy, positive emotion that has the power to create an energizing situation. Frustration, on the other hand, is a low-energy, negative emotion that will sap energy if allowed to linger. Emotions can be classified within an emotional quadrant involving both positive and negative elements and both high- and low-energy elements (Figure 6-1).

Low Energy	**High Energy**	
Relaxed Content Peaceful Tranquil In control	Excited Vigorous Engaged Confident Invigorated Challenged Patient Optimistic	**Positive**
Depressed Exhausted Concerned Agitated Fearful	Anxious Resentful Angry Bored Impatient Pessimistic Defensive	**Negative**

Figure 6-1

The four quadrants of emotion identified in Figure 6-1, and the common emotions associated with each area, are identified as follows:

- *Positive, high energy*: This quadrant represents the ideal emotional state for optimal athletic performance. It is characterised by high levels of energy, confidence, and enthusiasm, and can result in the high-energy flow state characteristic of optimal performance. The positive feelings associated with this state also encourage the mental toughness needed to consistently perform at a high level.
- *Positive, low energy*: This quadrant represents the ideal recovery state. The emotions in this quadrant can create energy, representing the ideal low-energy flow state required for recovery. While these low-energy emotions are not ideal for performance, the moods associated with this state create the necessary conditions for ideal recovery. Therefore, a key element of any recovery strategy is to engage in activities that encourage the emotions and states associated with this quadrant. These activities are likely to be very individualized and initially will be developed on a trial-and-error basis, but over time they will provide the athlete with the tools for developing appropriate recovery strategies.
- *Negative, high energy*: Although this quadrant represents a high-energy state, the negative emotions generated do not provide for the degree of control and stability required for consistently high performance. Very few athletes can perform consistently in this quadrant. Even if some athletes are occasionally able to perform well when they are within this quadrant, they will be unable to cope in the long-term with the energy-sapping consequences. This situation makes consistent high performance unlikely. Although it is not an ideal performance quadrant, all athletes will likely enter this quadrant at some time. It is important to identify times when negative high energy occurs, as well as the causes. Once these causes are identified, strategies and rituals can be set up to re-enter the positive high-energy quadrant (refer to Chapter 8). Doing so is the key to Pillar 5, where emotional strategies are developed that enable the athlete to cope with emotional stressors.
- *Negative, low energy*: This low-energy state does not promote recovery, as the negative emotions associated with this quadrant consistently sap energy. They set off a series of reactions that affect recovery on an emotional, psychological, and physical level. The emotions associated with this quadrant are among the most detrimental to overall health, and therefore performance as well. Continued time in this quadrant is highly likely to lead to many of the indicators of underrecovery.

Optimizing Performance and Recovery With the Quadrant

The essential aims of this pillar are to optimize performance and recovery:

- When athletes train and try to build capacity, they should attempt to spend as much of their time as possible in the positive, high-energy quadrant.

- When athletes are trying to recover, they should spend as much time as possible in the positive, low-energy quadrant.
- Athletes should spend as little time as possible in the negative portions of the quadrant.
- When they find themselves in the negative side, athletes should acknowledge the situation and try to find the cause. Doing so can then help in developing strategies to minimize the future effects of the stressors.

The Importance of Goals

The importance of goals is outlined in Pillar 1 (refer to Chapter 4). Goals have the ability to enhance time spent in the positive portions of the quadrant. Well-planned and challenging goals have the capacity to energize, invigorate, and engage an athlete while he is pursuing the goal. All of these states are characteristic of the positive, high-energy state required for optimal performance. After the goals are achieved, they contribute to a relaxed, contented feeling, leaving the athlete happy in the knowledge that the key tasks of the day have been achieved. These states are characteristic of the positive, low-energy states required for effective recovery. In both cases, the achievement of well-planned and challenging goals can significantly contribute to the mindset required for both optimal performance and optimal recovery.

Belief Systems Affect Mood State

A person's outlook on life, beliefs, and the way in which he explains any success or lack of success greatly affects the way he acts and behaves. The intricate relationships among physical, psychological, and emotional performance are outlined in Chapter 1. Everyone has experienced situations in which they have been relaxed and positive and seen how this state can positively affect all aspects of their lives. Similarly, everyone has probably experienced times when they have had a negative outlook and seen the detrimental effects this mood had on all aspects of their lives. Optimizing performance and recovery involves trying to create the necessary conditions to ensure that athletes stay in the positive half of the quadrant. Doing so involves maximizing the benefits of positive emotions and minimizing the debilitating effects of negative emotions. One key in this process is to examine an athlete's belief system and the effects it has on his emotions.

The way people frame their experiences greatly influences the way in which they react. A person's response to all experiences is affected by his internal system of beliefs, the majority of which have developed over time. While some people frame the vast majority of experiences in the positive, others will frame similar experiences in the negative. Therefore, similar experiences can have profoundly different effects on different people. The meaning a person gives to different situations will greatly affect his responses to the situation, and greatly influence whether the situation can be an energy giver or an energy sapper. The key to the Performance Lifestyle is to frame as many experiences as possible in the positive, which will facilitate optimal recovery. By framing experiences in the positive, athletes are given more choices in the way they deal with situations, which reduces the energy-sapping effects of negativity.

The Nature of Reality

What is reality? While the answer to this question may seem obvious, ask a group of people about any event and you will see that everyone has his own perception of reality. Indeed, many sports panel shows are built around sportswriters' perceptions of "reality," a reality that often differs from that of the viewer. Just ask any expert who is the greatest baseball player ever or who will win the next soccer World Cup, and you will see a whole host of attitudes and interpretations of the same events. Events are just events, and they can be seen as part of an objective world. What changes is a person's actual picture of the events, his subjective or inner world. This reality is created by the beliefs and thoughts the person brings to these events. Therefore, what a person calls reality is often tinged with his beliefs, values, perceptions, and thoughts.

During each day, an athlete will have to face a large number of different situations, each of which has the power to create energy or sap energy. What affect these situations have will largely be influenced by the individual's unique perception of reality.

Consider the following example: The head coach has been in his office since 7:00 a.m. watching game tape and thinks he sees a weakness in the opposition. He decides to get a cup of coffee before he sets about scripting plays for the day's practice. On his way down to the break room, he is picturing the plays in his head. He walks by two players, both of whom say, "Hi, Coach," but he is oblivious to them and doesn't reply:

- Player 1 thinks, "Something's up with Coach. Maybe something at home. Anyway we'll see him this afternoon."
- Player 2 thinks, "Coach totally ignored me. He must think I played badly on Saturday. Perhaps I'm not starting this coming Saturday."

Neither of these players has hit on the actual reality. While this scenario may not be a problem for player 1, for player 2 the morning could easily become a succession of self-doubting thoughts that will sap energy and compromise performance and recovery.

Clearly, a person's perceptions of reality may not be accurate and will be affected by his beliefs, thoughts, and emotions at any one time. A key to the Performance Lifestyle is to identify situations that sap energy and, if necessary, challenge the perception of reality to diffuse these situations.

Be Proactive

The need to take action was emphasized in Pillar 1 (refer to Chapter 4). Action is similarly vital in this pillar. Sitting back and complaining about situations will take athletes into the negative domain. While it is important for athletes to be able to identify areas that they need to address, it is equally important that they then take action to rectify the situation. Remember that knowledge without action is the same as not knowing. Therefore, once situations that result in negative emotions are identified, action needs to be taken to remedy the situation as best as possible. This pillar enables athletes to identify areas that need attention, and outlines methods by which the athlete can work on these areas. However, as always, these methods will only be successful if the athletes are proactive and take action.

The Explanatory Style—Optimism or Pessimism

How a person explains his success or failure greatly affects his mood states and his ability to stay positive. Much of a person's belief system is framed by the way in which he explains successes and failures—also called the person's explanatory style. Optimists tend to look at events, both successes and failures, in a way that maximizes positive emotion, while pessimists look at the same events and explain them in a way that develops negative emotions. The Performance Lifestyle is about building an optimistic outlook and avoiding pessimism wherever possible. Whether a person looks at events optimistically or pessimistically depends upon three key areas, which together explain the person's explanatory style:

- Permanence
- Pervasiveness
- Personalization

Permanence

Optimists believe that any setback is a temporary experience. They use sentences like, "I just had a bad day," "They got lucky," and "They won't beat us again," to explain any setbacks, which are usually seen as temporary. Pessimists, on the other hand, explain similar setbacks using statements such as "They're better than us," "I'm not much good," and "We'll never beat them." These statements suggest that the reasons for the setback are permanent rather than temporary. These explanatory styles can result in significantly different psychological profiles. While optimists recover quickly from setbacks and can recover their energy and motivation to move on, pessimists will often ruminate over events, which results in a helpless attitude that hinders recovery and subsequent action.

In successful situations, the reverse is often the case. Optimists will often explain success through permanence. For example, they will say, "I'm good at this game" or "I always play well in the big event." Pessimists will often explain success as a temporary feature. For example, they will say, "I got lucky today," "I played well today," or "My opponent was not playing his best." The difference in the permanence-related elements of explanatory style can significantly affect an athlete's emotional state.

Pervasiveness

Pervasiveness refers to the degree to which a failure in one area can affect other areas. For example, a golfer may be having trouble with his putting, but the rest of his game may be going well. An optimistic attitude would be to say, "My putting is a little off today, but the rest of my game is great. If I keep that going, my putting will come." For this golfer, putting is seen as a single part of the game, and poor performance in that area is not allowed to pervade the other elements of the game. A pessimist, on the other hand, might reply with a pervasive statement, such as, "My play is lousy today." In this simple change of explanation, poor performance in one element of the game has been allowed to affect all other parts of the game, even though the other elements were going well. The different effects of these styles are self-evident, yet many athletes will use the pervasive style of explanation even if doing so is clearly illogical. Athletes should try to avoid pervasiveness when explaining bad situations.

When explaining success, the reverse is true. Consider a golfing scenario in which putting is going well. An optimist will explain this situation with a pervasiveness that affects all areas, using statements such as, "I'm a great golfer." Pessimists, on the other hand, will isolate the putting with statements such as, "I'm good at putting." Athletes should try to use pervasiveness when explaining good situations.

Personalization

A pessimist will always explain a poor performance by personalizing it and putting the blame on himself. He will explain a good performance by externalizing it, saying the cause was something outside his control. On the other hand, an optimist will explain a poor performance by externalizing it and a good performance by personalizing it.

When a pessimist does well, he will say things such as, "My opponent had an off day," or "Luck was on my side," thereby externalizing the reasons. An optimist will personalize the situation with statements such as, "I'm a great player," and "They can't keep up with me." On the other hand, when a pessimist does badly, he will use phrases such as "I was not good enough today," or "My skills let me down," thereby personalising the reason. The optimist, on the other hand, externalizes the failure with reasons such as, "They just had a good day," or "They won't be so lucky next time." Again, these explanatory styles have the capacity to significantly alter emotions.

To assist both performance and recovery, an athlete should always try to be an optimist in explaining both success and failure. He should use optimistic phrases whenever possible, both during performance and throughout life. Doing so will enhance both performance and recovery, and also have the benefit of enhancing his quality of life by creating an optimistic outlook that will reduce the likelihood of depression.

Changing the Belief System

Earlier in this chapter, the nature of reality was examined, including how an athlete's version of reality will be created by the belief systems he holds. Additionally, the need for an optimistic outlook on life and events, both within and outside the athletic arena, was stressed. A key in creating an optimistic outlook is to examine and, if necessary, change the athlete's belief system. Remember, an optimist will explain any setbacks as temporary, nonpervasive, and external. The ability to be optimistic requires the development of appropriate belief systems and, if necessary, requires the challenging and changing of the athlete's existing belief systems.

Unfortunately, many of an athlete's belief systems are being reinforced on a daily basis by self-talk, which is the constant dialogue that goes on in an athlete's mind—what can be termed "the inner critic." If an athlete was told by a fan that he is a poor athlete, a poor friend, or a poor teammate only looking after his own interests, he would likely argue quite vehemently with the fan to counter these accusations. However, many athletes are being told similar things every day by their own inner critics.

Consider the following situation: An athlete misses a penalty shot in soccer. His inner voice says, "What was that? You don't deserve to be on the team. You've let all your teammates down. You're a hopeless penalty taker." Unfortunately, when these statements come from their inner voice, many athletes simply accept them as true. Unlike in the earlier example in which the athlete will argue with the fan, he simply accepts these statements, regardless of whether they are based on any rational facts. Clearly, if such statements are accepted on a regular basis, then it will be difficult to maintain an optimistic outlook. Pessimism may dominate, along with its associated drain on energy.

A key to remaining optimistic, and thus in the positive part of the quadrant, is to change these beliefs and minimize the effect of the inner critic. The Performance Lifestyle uses two techniques to achieve this objective:

- The ABCD system invented by noted psychologist Martin Seligman (2003) is a powerful tool with which to change a person's beliefs.

- The second system was outlined by Paul McKenna (2004) and is a powerful tool with which to develop a positive optimistic outlook by marginalizing the inner voice.

The ABCD System

The general comments section of the daily log will have developed an athlete's ability to identify the most common negative emotions he is feeling. By using this tool, the athlete should have started to get an idea of the main problem thoughts he is experiencing. The ABCD tool focuses on identifying and changing the belief systems that underpin these thoughts. The good news is that these belief systems do not have to be permanent. By performing the exercises in this pillar, the athlete will be able to change these belief systems and therefore increase the likelihood of remaining in the positive side of the quadrant. Unfounded or irrational beliefs lead to energy loss and additional stress. Through the work in Pillar 2, the athlete should have become aware of his problematic emotions (refer to Chapter 5). The next step is to identify, challenge, and change the beliefs that are causing negativity via the ABCD system. Figure 6-2 shows an example of the ABCD system and Figure 6-3 presents a completed example of the ABCD exercise outlined in the following section.

Changing Beliefs—Creating Optimism

A—What has happened that is affecting your emotions? What emotions are you feeling and how are they affecting your moods?

B—What beliefs are these feelings caused by?

C—What are the consequences of these beliefs?

D—Dispute these beliefs.

Figure 6-2

In the ABCD system:

- "A" represents the *activating* event, which could be a competition, the coach shouting, a failed putt in golf, etc. This act initiates the problem.
- "B" represents the athlete's *beliefs*. For example, when the coach shouts at the athlete, the belief may be, "He hates me," or "I'm no good at this game." This belief is at the root of the problem.
- "C" represents the *consequences*. The consequences in this case could be that the athlete goes into his shell and sulks after being shouted at, which results in him concentrating on the negativity and making more mistakes..
- "D" represents the athlete actually *disputing* the belief and arguing with himself about the beliefs. By challenging the beliefs, he will often find that the beliefs are unfounded, and that they can be changed. If the beliefs are changed, they will greatly reduce the negative consequences of future similar actions.

When disputing the belief systems, the athlete should actively address the following questions:

- Is the belief really true?
- How do I know that the belief is really true?
- Where is the evidence?

As the athlete does this exercise, he will probably find that his beliefs are not based on fact, but simply on his interpretation of issues. As he continues, he will start to question, then challenge, and then disagree with his beliefs. He can then replace these beliefs with positive statements.

This exercise can be particularly effective if the athlete has someone else to argue with—externalizing his inner critic. The other person will present the athlete's beliefs and the athlete will counter him. If the athlete can find someone he trusts to do this exercise with, it can be an especially effective.

Marginalize the Inner Critic and Build the Inner Coach

Unfortunately, an athlete's greatest critic is often his own inner critic. This self-criticism runs through the athlete's head and can be one of the biggest challenges to a positive outlook. The ABCD system is a valuable tool when trying to change these beliefs. As a second defense against the inner critic, the Performance Lifestyle recommends that the athlete seek to marginalize the inner critic by utilizing the technique outlined in Figure 6-4.

This technique is based on changing the psychological profile of the inner voice and is based on the fact that the influence of the inner voice will be closely linked to the perception of its authority. Imagine that you have gone to a coaches' conference

Changing Beliefs—Creating Optimism

A—What has happened that is affecting your emotions? What emotions are you feeling and how are they affecting your moods?

Our soccer game came down to a penalty shootout. I came forward to take the first one and missed. I'm feeling ashamed, guilty, and annoyed. I've been in a bad mood for days, grumpy, and irritable.

B—What beliefs are these feelings caused by?

I believe I've let the team down. I was the first one up, was supposed to be the best, and I missed. How can I be a good soccer player if I can't take a penalty and score. It's because of me that we lost.

C—What are the consequences of these beliefs?

I can't face my coach and my teammates. I now doubt my soccer ability and don't know if the sport's for me. I've been feeling low ever since the game.

D—Dispute these beliefs.

I was the one who scored two goals to take us to extra time. I must be pretty good to do that. The team said how well I played in regular time and during the extra time.

Yes, I missed, but so did three others. It wasn't all down to me.

Coach wanted me to take the first one to give us a good start, so he must have thought I was good.

Their keeper was on form that day. He just guessed right, and that won't happen too often.

Even the best players in the world miss penalties now and again.

Figure 6-3

Whenever you hear the inner voice criticizing you, focus on your perception of the inner critic:

- Imagine that you have a volume control and turn the volume down a little.
- Imagine that you have a button that changes the sound of the voice to that of a cartoon character like Donald Duck (or any other ridiculous voice).

Now listen to your inner critic. How seriously are you now taking what it is saying? Even if you cannot stop the inner critic, you can at least marginalize it and reduce its impact. From now on, every time you hear the inner critic, hear it in these terms with the volume down and the cartoon voice.

Figure 6-4

and someone gets up to talk about building confidence in a team. As he gets up and starts to talk, his voice is that of a cartoon character and is at a very low volume. How much credence are you going to give to this speaker? This scenario is the foundation upon which this technique is built.

The reverse needs to be done for the inner coach. The inner coach is the praise the athlete gives himself and these thoughts can positively affect performance. Complements, positive coaching tips, etc., are all very useful elements of the inner coach. This feedback will ideally be delivered by a powerful and well-respected voice. Therefore, with this voice, an athlete needs to use the voice of someone he feels has great authority and assign this voice to his inner coach. Similarly, when the athlete turns up the volume, this voice is given even greater authority. Athletes can use the following techniques to develop their inner coach:

- The athlete should identify times when the inner coach is working.
- He can then turn up the volume so that he is getting positive affirmations as often as possible.
- He should assign the voice of someone he really respects to this voice.

Be in Control—Avoid Learned Helplessness

A result of a pessimistic attitude in the face of any setbacks can be a state called learned helplessness. This state is characterized by a feeling that whatever a person does, he cannot affect the things that are bothering him. Rather than developing a proactive attitude, where the athlete actively tries to address the causes of setbacks, inactivity becomes the norm. Martin Seligman (2006) links this state with depression and outlines severe repercussions for people who stay in this state for extended periods. While athletes may not encounter these clinical problems of depression, etc., the capacity of a pessimistic explanatory style does have the capacity to negatively affect both performance and recovery. In contrast, the optimistic style initiates bouncing back from adversity and responding with positive actions. Key issues can be addressed via the use of effective rituals (refer to Chapter 7).

An empowered athlete is able to make quality decisions in all aspects of the Performance Lifestyle. The athlete must always focus on aspects of his life that are under his control. Doing so allows for positive actions to be taken that can directly enhance the Performance Lifestyle. Focusing on aspects outside his control is likely to result in negative moods, as he will be unable to influence these things. Pillar 4 identifies how an athlete can use rituals to positively affect any aspects that his self-awareness highlights as in need of development (refer to Chapter 7).

Go to the Movies—Building the Self-Image

An athlete's performance and recovery ability will be affected by his self-image. In any activity, he will only be as successful as he allows himself to be. To allow himself to be successful, a positive self-image is vital. The ABCD and inner-voice activities will help build this self-image. Another particularly effective strategy is to supplement these activities with the use of the movies activity used in Pillar 1 (refer to Figure 4-2).

Just as all of the senses were used to develop a quality image of the athletes achieving their goals, athletes should develop quality movies of themselves being successful in all of the activities they highlight as needing attention. These positive images can be used regularly to develop an athlete's positive self-image, which will contribute to positivity, and thus to recovery and subsequent performance. In addition to the mental movies, real film clips of successful performances are a great tool in developing a positive mindset. Athletes should be encouraged to collect film clips of themselves performing well, whether during training or competition. With the availability of low-cost video editing software, these films can be effectively edited into a series of motivational video montages that an athlete can use whenever needed.

Frame Everything Positively—Use Positive Statements

The way people talk to themselves greatly influences the way they are received, and subsequently their mood states. Consider questions and statements such as, "Why can't I do this?" "Why do things always go wrong?" "Why don't I ever perform at the big event?" These questions are all negatively framed and suggest a lack of ability to cope with key situations.

Consider the following statement, which is made by a tennis player: "I just can't seem to master the volley." This tennis player, by framing his frustration at his lack of progress with the volley shot, immediately produces a negative feedback. By framing his self-talk in this way, he is saying to himself that the volley is a key shot in tennis and that he is unable to perform this skill. Compare this player with another player who is having similar problems with the volley, but asks himself, "How can I make this shot work more effectively?" This question suggests that the shot can work, that a number of answers exist, and that the athlete is able to come up with the answers. While the first athlete uses a negative framework, the latter uses a positive one. Therefore, the latter athlete is increasing his chances of both staying in the positive quadrant and of actually mastering the task.

Statements and questions need to be framed positively. Questions like, "How can I best solve this?" and "How many solutions can I come up with to this problem?" are far more likely to result in positive-quadrant mood states. Therefore, the athlete is more likely to optimize both performance and recovery than if he used negatively framed questions such as "Why can't I do this?" As an example, two golfers approach the eighteenth green, which is surrounded on three sides by water. Figure 6-5 presents their inner statements.

	Athlete 1	**Athlete 2**
Statement	Stay out of the water	Lay it up next to the flag
Area of focus	The water	The green
Consequence	Mind focuses on the water, not the green	Mind focuses on the green, not the water
Result	Ball goes into the water	Ball stays on the green
Energy result	Energy lost	Energy conserved

Figure 6-5

In Figure 6-5, athlete 1 frames the situation with negative statements, which results in poor performance, while athlete 2 frames it positively. Similarly, the example in Figure 6-6 shows how two athletes frame an additional videotape session. Again, simply framing an activity positively creates a completely different outcome.

The team has just finished a physically tough practice and the players now know that they will have to review a tape of that practice, even though nobody really wants to. Consider the two reactions to this scenario:

- Athlete 1: This is just coach getting back at us. It won't be much use, but I'll just grin and bear it.
- Athlete 2: It's tough, but at least I'll get the chance to look at my blocking technique.

Athlete 1 frames the experience negatively. During the review session, he is likely to feel bored, frustrated, or even angry—all negative feelings. These feelings will sap energy and increase fatigue.

Athlete 2 has framed it positively and is more likely to stay in the positive quadrant, resulting in fewer energy leaks and a greater degree of recovery.

Figure 6-6

The Importance of Being Surrounded by Positive People

Personal relationships have a huge impact on whether athletes view experiences as positive or negative. An athlete's views and beliefs can be greatly influenced by the people that surround him. Everyone has probably experienced people whose presence inspires them and places them immediately in a positive frame of mind. On the other hand, everyone has also experienced people who are constantly in a negative frame of mind and are always criticizing and complaining, and then experienced how negative this environment can be on a person's energy levels.

A simple strategy to create a positive environment is to be surrounded by positive people. The environment created within the training arena can greatly affect the productivity of any training program, and can create the supportive and motivational environment needed for optimal recovery and performance. Coaches need to constantly note the positive and negative behaviors of all people within the training environment, as everyone has the ability to affect energy positively and negatively. This training must include coaching staff, athletes, and support staff, and needs to evaluate these effects on an individual and group basis. This evaluation needs to be ongoing, as a multitude of factors can influence a person's attitudes. Where negative tendencies are identified, they need to be addressed quickly, before they negatively affect the performance and recovery of a larger group.

Seek Out the Gratifications

People will have a number of pleasures and gratifications over the course of their lives. It is important to determine the difference between these categories, as they have distinctly different effects on long-term emotional fitness. Pleasures are short-term and, while they bring short-term positive emotions, these emotions can often be dissipated rapidly and leave behind a craving. Eating a bar of chocolate is an example. As a person eats chocolate, it brings him pleasure, albeit pleasure that peaks in the first bite and then dissipates. However, once the event is over, the positive effects will disappear quite rapidly, and indeed can often be replaced by negative feelings (e.g., regret and guilt). Activities such as binge eating, drinking alcohol, watching TV, hanging around with friends, etc., can be thought of as pleasures. While pleasures are important, it is also important that an athlete's life does not solely revolve around these pleasures. A feature of many pleasures is that to recreate the positivity, it is often necessary to recreate the pleasure. This fact is part of the problem with alcohol and drugs, which create very short-term highs that are often followed by periods of negative emotions and the need for another dose of the "pleasure." This scenario creates a whole host of negative emotions, which ultimately can only be alleviated by the dose of pleasure, which is ultimately contributing to the problem. It is this constant need for the pleasure that creates addiction patterns.

Gratifications, on the other hand, have the capacity to build positive emotion for a much longer period of time. They can often be linked with activities that contribute to the greater good. Working hard and achieving good grades is an example of a gratification. An almost contradictory feature of gratifications is that, at the time, the activity will be challenging, involve effort, and may not be initially pleasurable, such as a really challenging conditioning session. During these activities, the individual may be attracted to pleasures. For example, the student working hard to achieve high grades may feel that he would prefer to be hanging around the mall with other youngsters. In the long-term, however, the achievement will bring around more positive emotion than that experienced by the individuals who only involved themselves with the pleasures. In many cases, sports participation is a gratification that provides long-term achievement associated with the greater good (i.e., committing effort to the success of the team).

Life balance is an important concept for developing the low-energy, positive mood states characteristic of optimal recovery. It is important that the athlete can commit to activities away from athletics that also provide gratification, and provide this life balance, which addresses their basic needs as identified in Chapter 4. The lifestyle profile used in Chapter 5 can assist the athlete and coach in identifying whether the athlete is managing his time and energy in a way that is conducive to life balance and recovery.

This need for gratifications away from athletics is especially important for professional athletes, who often have considerable spare time and do not naturally participate in the type of activities that produce gratifications. In some cases, this time is spent seeking pleasures to provide excitement. In these cases, activities such as gambling may become a problem. Education is crucial in attaining this life balance, as athletes need to be clear about its importance to performance and recovery. Additionally, they need to be empowered to actually undertake the activities that will provide the gratification they require.

Summary

- A person's outlook on life will greatly affect his performance and recovery.
- Emotions can be classified into an emotional quadrant, and athletes should try to stay in the positive half of the grid for as much time as possible.
- Reality is shaped by a person's experiences, thoughts, and beliefs.
- An optimistic outlook is conducive to higher levels of performance and recovery.
- People are able to change their outlook by changing their belief systems. The ABCD system and marginalizing the inner critic allow us to do this.
- Control is important in developing positivity.
- An athlete should always be working to build his self-image through activities such as mental movies, positive framing, surrounding himself with positive people, and seeking out gratifications.

7

Pillar 4—
The Power of Rituals

"We are what we repeatedly do.
Excellence then is not an act but a habit."

—Aristotle

At many times throughout this book, the need to take action is stressed. Action is fundamental to creating the Performance Lifestyle, allowing athletes to make the decisions and implement the changes that lead to enhanced recovery and performance. But how can athletes most effectively take action and, when needed, permanently change behavior in an energy-efficient way?

Positive rituals lie at the heart of the Performance Lifestyle, as they represent the most important way of taking positive action and are the key way of positively modifying an athlete's lifestyle. While self-discipline is so lauded in athletics, in the Performance Lifestyle self-discipline is superseded by positive rituals. In itself, self-discipline suggests sacrifice, and while sacrifice is important in many instances, it also brings with it a negative connotation. It implies that the athlete is concerned with avoidance, which again has a negative connotation. When the aim is to avoid doing something, the focus is naturally placed on the action that needs to be avoided, which increases the difficulty in avoiding it, in essence glorifying the very thing that the athlete is trying to avoid. This scenario has the effect of creating energy leaks, which are detrimental to recovery. Rituals, on the other hand, work on the positive side of the equation, focusing on the positive action to be taken, rather than on the negative action to be avoided.

Rituals—The Low-Energy Alternative

Not doing something, as implied by the notion of self-discipline, is a negatively framed statement that contradicts the need for positivity, as outlined in Pillar 3 (refer to Chapter 6). This type of framing requires a great deal of energy to be expended in the "avoidance" of an action. Psychologists also believe that the mind finds it difficult to differentiate between the positive and negative. When an athlete is telling himself, "Don't eat poorly," the mind interprets this statement as "Eat poorly," and a great deal of self-discipline and energy is expended.

Acting by ritual, on the other hand, expends very little energy. Considering the things that people do every day, it is likely that many actions occur with little if any active thought—they are rituals that people undertake. For example, when an athlete wakes up in the morning, he probably does the same thing every day (e.g., go to the toilet, shower, brush his teeth), and all of this activity requires very little thought or effort. Rituals work in a very similar way. Every time a person performs an action it becomes engrained in his subconscious and the body finds it easier to repeat the pattern. As people perform these actions on a regular basis, they become a part of a daily routine—a ritual. The key to rituals is that they require little conscious thought and are ideal in terms of reducing energy expenditure. However, they do take time to develop, and need to be actively pursued in the early stages of development.

Positive Rituals

Rituals should always be positively framed and involve actions that contribute to recovery and general health. They should involve a "movement toward" attitude, rather than an "avoidance" attitude. For example, the statement "I'm not going to eat chocolate for a month" reveals an avoidance attitude, implying the need for great self-discipline. Remember, people who frame activities in this way actually focus on the very thing they are trying to avoid. Instead, rituals are positive activities where the focus is on carrying out an action that makes a positive change. In the chocolate example, had a ritual been framed in a positive and action-oriented way, such as "I take a piece of fruit with me to work and eat it on my break," it is far more likely that the person will be successful.

When Should Rituals Be Used?

The great thing about rituals is their low energy requirement. Working through the first few pillars should have identified the athlete's goals, built his awareness of his capacity and recovery, and identified the beliefs that he needs to change to remain positive. Rituals will be a key method by which the athlete will achieve many of these goals.

Rituals therefore need to be utilized at many times during the day and involve both athletic and nonathletic activities. For example, the athlete needs to refuel as soon as possible following a workout or other activity. A positive ritual would be for the athlete to identify an appropriate refuelling food and ensure that he takes it with him to the workout and consumes it immediately after the workout finishes. While this task may require an active reminder the first few times, after a while it will become second nature and be established as a ritual that positively affects recovery. Rituals need to be used in all three domains of fitness and should provide the basic structure around which the Performance Lifestyle can be constructed.

The Progression of Ritualistic Actions

It is likely that an athlete will need to make a number of key lifestyle changes when working toward his optimal Performance Lifestyle. It is highly unlikely that an athlete will be able to make all of the required changes at once. Rather than making radical total life changes, a progressive move is needed to reach toward the optimal Performance Lifestyle. An athlete must find a level of progression that he can live with, yet provides benefits that are real and impact performance.

The first step is the prioritizing of the key areas of the lifestyle to address. The work in the self-awareness and goal-setting pillars should have identified key areas that the athlete needs to address. This information then forms the template of the plan. Once the key areas are identified, a small number of rituals can be developed that are designed to address key issues. The athlete should ensure that these rituals are attainable and should focus on no more than two or three rituals at any one time. Once these rituals are embedded into the lifestyle, then more can be progressively added. In this way, while each step may be small and very manageable, over time significant changes are embedded into an athlete's lifestyle.

Developing the Ritual

Figure 7-1 can be used to develop positive rituals that will form the foundation of the Performance Lifestyle. Doing so involves four key processes:

- Identifying the aspect of the athlete's lifestyle that is to be modified, usually based on the feedback from the self-awareness work
- Outlining the consequences of the problem
- Identifying what needs to be done, as specifically as possible
- Outlining exactly how to achieve this objective—the precise ritual to be performed

Figure 7-2 outlines how the ritual-setting sheet can be used for an athlete who has identified the need to refuel effectively immediately after exercise.

Ritual Setting

What is the problem?

What are the consequences of the problem?

What do you need to do?

Describe the ritual that you will follow.

Figure 7-1

Ritual Setting

What is the problem?
I have a late practice every Tuesday. Because of this schedule, when I get home I relax and try to go to sleep, so I don't eat until the next morning. In these cases, I will normally wake up in the middle of the night starving and just eat the easiest thing, normally biscuits. Alternatively, when I get home I try to make myself something to eat, which takes time. In this case, I then don't relax and can't get off to sleep for a long time.

What are the consequences of the problem?
I don't get a full night of sleep.
I feel guilty about eating poorly.
I don't get the quality nutrition I need to recover.
I don't feel recovered in the morning.

What do you need to do?
I need to eat immediately after training to maximize my recovery and to allow myself to relax and go to sleep when I get home.

Describe the ritual that you will follow.
I will prepare a meal and appropriate supplements prior to training. I will then take them with me to ensure that I take in an appropriate refuelling meal immediately after training.

Figure 7-2

Habits—Cure and Curse

While positive rituals are the preferred method by which many of the Performance Lifestyle aspects will be achieved due to their low energy requirements, negative rituals can cause problems. Rituals become habits, and some of an athlete's activities may be contributing to his lack of recovery. For example, the team may have a ritual of going for fast food immediately after training sessions. Doing so will considerably negate recovery, yet it may have developed into such a habit that it may be difficult to break at first. In developing self-awareness, it is important to identify aspects of the lifestyle that are contributing to the lack of recovery. The reasons for these behaviors then need to be identified, and new positive rituals engineered to counter the problem. The following steps need to be carried out:

- Identify the problem activity.
- Identify actions that are contributing to the problem. In doing this exercise, athletes may identify habits are contributing to the problem activity.
- Develop a new ritual that will help solve the problem, and then develop positive actions.

Summary

- Athletes need to take action to achieve their goals.
- Rituals are low-energy methods by which positive lifestyle changes can be affected. They are preferred over self-discipline, which suggests avoidance.
- The Performance Lifestyle is constructed around positive rituals.
- Rituals must always be positive and include an action toward a goal. They should never be framed in terms of avoidance.
- A small number of rituals should be developed at any one time.

8

Pillar 5— Build Capacity and Recover

"Sometimes it's important to work for that pot of gold. But other times it's essential to take time off and make sure that your most important decision in the day simply consists of choosing which color to slide down on the rainbow."

—Douglas Pagels

Previous chapters and pillars have illustrated how optimal performance and recovery depend upon the unique interaction among levels of stress, fatigue, and recovery in all three domains of fitness. To optimize performance, athletes need to develop their ability to tolerate multidimensional stress, and to facilitate recovery via proactive measures that address all of the key pillars. A unique feature of the Performance Lifestyle approach to enhancing recovery is that it involves activities that build capacity, in addition to activities designed to facilitate regeneration and recovery. Rather than simply employing methods that focus solely on enhancing recovery, the Performance Lifestyle focuses on building an athlete's capacity to tolerate stressors, thus reducing the negative effects of these stressors on performance. This two-pronged attack maximizes an athlete's recovery levels as well as his levels of performance.

Chapter 1 clearly illustrates the multidimensional nature of fitness and recovery, with total stress dependent upon the summation of stressors from all three domains, as well as the cybernetic link among these stressors. A key aspect of building a Performance Lifestyle involves building capacity and facilitating recovery in each domain. In this way, optimal recovery can be achieved. By increasing capacity, tolerance for stress in that domain will increase, simultaneously enhancing the recovery process. It is important to note, however, that this enhanced capacity will be specific to the training undertaken. Therefore, for optimal effectiveness, all domains have to be developed. In addition, activities must be targeted at each athlete's unique sources of stressors, which will have been identified in earlier pillars. By carefully manipulating recovery activities, athletes can ensure that the ability to handle and recover from these stressors is optimized. This pillar, therefore, is constructed to actively build capacity in each domain, while also actively regenerating and controlling overall stress levels.

Applying Universal Training Principles

When building capacity, the traditional training principles such as specificity, overload, progression, and recovery, which are characteristic of physical training, can be applied to all domains. Capacity development should be specific to the stress tolerance needed. Similarly, a level of overload is needed to build this enhanced capacity. The principle of overload requires an ever-increasing level of controlled stress be placed on an athlete if he is to continue to make training gains. Therefore, recovery within a Performance Lifestyle must not be seen merely as an avoidance of stress. The universal training principles are the foundation of all physical-training programs, but unfortunately are not often applied to the psychological and emotional domains. It is important to remember that high levels of controlled training stress are often needed in training programs. Indeed, athletes simply cannot reach their full potential without that stress. However, the stress needs to be controlled and subjected to careful planning, as outlined later in this chapter. One of the key premises of the Performance Lifestyle approach is not always to reduce stress (as doing so is not always possible or even effective), but instead to increase the capacity to tolerate stress. Via the work in Pillar 2, the athlete should have identified key areas of performance to target, which will provide the focus for the capacity-building programs (refer to Chapter 5). During the program, the recovery-training log can then be used to monitor how the athlete is responding to these stressors, and appropriate modifications can be made to optimize performance.

It has been consistently stressed how total fitness is concerned with the cybernetic relationships among the three domains of fitness—physical, psychological, and emotional. Therefore, to comply with this total fitness model, increased stress-tolerance capacity needs to occur in all three domains as well. Focusing on one domain to the detriment of others will always lead to less than optimal performance in the long term, creating a weak link in the total performance chain. Similarly, recovery and regeneration activities need to be undertaken in all domains.

Build Capacity and Regenerate

The key to this pillar of the Performance Lifestyle is to build capacity in all domains and then regenerate—again in all domains. Building capacity will require periodically high levels of stress, which should be carefully targeted at each athlete's areas of need.

However, all athletes have a certain tolerance for stress and a limited energy pool. Therefore, the development of capacity needs to be targeted at the individual. Athletes simply cannot train at high intensities (which are required for increased capacity) for extended periods of time. Therefore, training is most effective when the focus is on quality and not quantity. Once training is complete, the key for the athlete is to regenerate. Again, this regeneration needs to take place in all three domains of fitness. Indeed, the success of this approach will be intricately linked to the regeneration work carried out. If regeneration is not addressed or is insufficient, training progress will never be optimal, regardless of the complexity of the program.

Regeneration needs to occur in all domains and needs to be related to the types and levels of stress being experienced. In other words, regeneration needs to be targeted in both type and volume. In this way, periods of high training volume, such as in training camps, should instigate a greater number of regenerative initiatives. These initiatives can also be targeted at the type of fatigue (e.g., neural-based exercises will require neural-based regenerative activities, such as contrast showers) (Figure 8-1), as well as the quantity of fatigue.

Types of Physical Fatigue and Appropriate Recovery Strategies		
Type of Fatigue	**Causes**	**Strategies**
Metabolic	High training volume Metabolic conditioning (aerobic and anaerobic) Multiple training sessions	Sleep Refuelling nutrition Contrast bathing Active recovery (cool down) Pool recovery session Sleep (deep sleep)
Tissue damage	Plyometrics Heavy eccentric loads Contact sports	Nutrition Cold baths Compression clothing Pool recovery session Sleep (deep sleep)
Neural	High-intensity work Speed and agility work Strength and power training	Massage Cold baths Sleep (REM sleep)

Figure 8-1

A key benefit to accrue from the self-awareness pillar is the athlete's ability to identify periods of greater stress, as well as his typical sources of stress. Similarly, it will also develop his ability to identify times when his recovery may be less than optimal. Both scenarios represent a clear sign to increase the amount of recovery and regeneration work they are undertaking.

Building Capacity—The Interval Training Approach

Capacity in all domains is best built with short levels of intense activity, followed by periods of active regeneration. This training method is similar to the interval approach to training favored by many track coaches, whereby short periods of intense training are interspersed with recovery periods of varying durations.

The Performance Lifestyle approach therefore involves two elements:

- *Active capacity development*: Capacity is developed in the three dimensions and targeted at the key areas within each dimension.
- *Active regeneration*: Activities are undertaken that facilitate recovery in all three dimensions.

A successful performance program should involve the careful planning and programming of both of these elements. Unfortunately, while physical training is usually carefully planned, training for psychological and emotional fitness is not, and is often lacking in an athlete's performance program. Similarly, recovery and regeneration are often overlooked—serious omissions if programs are to be optimally effective. In such situations, consistent optimal performance can never be achieved.

Active Engagement

The approach of the Performance Lifestyle involves training smarter rather than training longer. All training should have a defined purpose and involve short periods of very active engagement. Once these activities are done, they should be followed by periods of active regeneration. In this way, the results from all training activities can be maximized, while the regeneration activities allow for the appropriate adaptations to occur and for the body to remobilize in preparation for the next dose of training stress.

An important aspect of this process is the delineation of loads—that is, how much training will be allocated to each domain, and to each variable within that domain. For example, in a training week, how much work will be allocated to physical elements such as speed and strength, psychological elements such as confidence and visualization, and to emotional elements such as self-control and relationship development? In general, three types of loads can be identified:

- *Stimulation loads*: A load that develops a physical capacity
- *Maintenance loads*: A load that maintains a physical capacity
- *Detraining loads*: A load that results in decreased performance

If the physical dimension is examined as an example, many sports require that a huge number of fitness parameters be developed. In basketball, for example, athletes need to have speed, agility, strength, power, endurance, etc. It is impossible to develop all of these fitness variables at any one time, and so stimulation loads are normally assigned to the specific fitness variables that need to be developed at any given time. However, an athlete needs to ensure that the other fitness variables are assigned loads that will ensure that they are maintained. Stimulation loads, or loads where the aim is to develop performance, are significantly higher than the loads required to maintain performance (maintenance loads). However, maintenance is crucial at all times. The "use it or lose it" maxim is true, and loads need to be allocated that at least maintain fitness and do not result in detraining. Luckily, the requirements for maintenance loads are significantly lower than for stimulation, and many parameters can be maintained with the allocation of maintenance loads. This assignment of loads is fundamental to the concept of periodization, which is in itself vital to optimal performance.

Active Disengagement

While the term itself may appear to be an oxymoron, active disengagement is fundamental to any recovery lifestyle. No human being can remain engaged for any extended length of time without paying severe consequences. Thus, once engagement ceases, athletes need to come up with various rituals and strategies that provide for recovery on an emotional, physical, and psychological basis. Unfortunately, active disengagement is often the most overlooked part of any training program. As stated many times in this book, if athletes do not recover, they will never perform optimally.

A number of disengagement and regeneration strategies are outlined in this chapter. However, given the individual nature of stress, fatigue, and subsequent recovery, the effectiveness of each will be highly individualized. Each athlete, therefore, needs to experiment with these methods and establish which work for him. Once the preferred methods are identified, they can be developed into appropriate rituals to ensure recovery and regeneration in all fitness domains.

Recovery Needs to Be Related to Engagement

As self-awareness develops, so does the power to evaluate the levels of stress and the sources of that stress. In times of high stress, whatever the source, an increased need for specific disengagement and recovery-based activities will be present. For example, during training camps, physical rituals, such as those outlined later in this chapter, need to be increased. Similarly, due to the high levels of psychological engagement, psychological-recovery strategies need to be increased. At all times, the recovery strategies must be in proportion to the level of engagement and targeted at the predominant types and sources of stress.

This principle is also true in relation to the nature of the stressor. Physical stressors, for example, can be predominantly physiological or neural. Depending upon the predominant stress, the preferred recovery strategy will differ.

Recovery Will Be Multidimensional

Any recovery strategy can work in a multidimensional way, promoting or possibly retarding physical, psychological, and emotional recovery. For example, low-intensity activities such as a gentle pool workout can provide for effective recovery in a number of domains. Physically, these workouts can increase the elimination of waste, promote the delivery of nutrients to the muscle, promote mobility, etc. Psychologically, they can provide for a break from traditional training routines and prevent boredom. Emotionally, they can enhance enjoyment and relaxation. When choosing strategies, it is important that athletes look at their effects in all domains and make appropriate choices based on this information. Ice baths, for example, may provide effective physical recovery for the majority of athletes, but may cause great anxiety for others, as some athletes will not enjoy the experience. In some instances, the psychological stress may outweigh the physical benefits and the process may retard rather than facilitate recovery. In these cases, the athlete needs to evaluate the net effectiveness of all strategies on a multidimensional basis. Again, the recovery log will facilitate this process.

The Effectiveness of Strategies Will Be Related to Disengagement

Whatever recovery strategy is chosen, the activity will not be fully effective unless total disengagement occurs. For example, during one pool workout an athlete may be focused not on the activity, but rather on the disagreement he just had with the coach. Therefore, while providing for some physical recovery, in this instance the psychological and emotional recovery is nonexistent, and overall stress levels are actually building as the athlete ruminates on this disagreement. Therefore, whatever regenerative activity is being undertaken, it is important to ensure that full disengagement occurs for optimal recovery. The psychological methods presented in this chapter provide detail on disengagement strategies.

Strategies Need to Be Individualized

As recovery will occur in a multidimensional domain, strategies need to be related not only to the type of activity, but also to the individual's perception of both the activity and his own needs. If 10 athletes were asked about their favorite recovery technique,

10 different answers would likely be given. For example, while massage may be popular with one individual, another may dislike massage. In this case, massage may provide for multidimensional recovery for one athlete, yet cause psychological stress for the other, which could counteract any physical gains from the massage.

Therefore, athletes need to develop their own individual routines and rituals. They also need to develop a range of rituals, as some activities may not always be available. For example, some athletes may like ice baths after a game. However, the facilities may not be available in some locations. Therefore, athletes need to have alternate strategies and may choose to use self-massage as an alternate recovery strategy.

Building Capacity and Regenerating

Outlined in the remainder of this chapter are guidelines for building capacity and regenerating. For ease of organization, the guidelines are classified into the three dimension of fitness. However, it is important to remember that many methods used will have the capacity to work in multiple domains, and their effects should not be seen in isolation. The example of massage is evidence of how a predominantly physical method can also work in the psychological and emotional domains.

THE PHYSICAL DOMAIN

Optimal physical performance will depend upon the precise interaction between the physical stressors required to enhance performance and regeneration. For optimal effectiveness, an athlete needs to develop his physical capacity, while at the same time controlling overall stress levels and providing for optimal regeneration and recovery.

Developing Physical Capacity

A well-designed training program is essential for optimal performance. However, a poorly designed program can also lead to underrecovery. Indeed, underrecovery can be traced to mistakes in the training process. Some of the most common training mistakes leading to underrecovery include the following:

- Recovery is neglected.
- Training demands are increased too rapidly.
- Workload is too high following a layoff.
- Excessive volume is used.
- Excessive high-intensity training is performed.
- Too much emphasis is placed on complex demands.
- Excessive competition is present.
- Biased training direction is evident (e.g., too much high-intensity power work).

It would be impossible to outline an appropriate training program for all athletes within this text, as it is well beyond the scope of the book. All training undertaken should be directed by a qualified strength and conditioning coach. If this situation is not feasible, follow a well-researched program such as the Performance Training system used by All-Pro Performance (www.allproperformance.co.uk), which adheres to the latest scientific information. When evaluating a program, the principles discussed in the following sections should be considered.

Follow a periodized year plan.

Periodization is a system in which the year is split into a number of cycles. In periodization terms, the year itself is the macrocycle. The year can then be broken down into specific phases, or mesocycles. These cycles can be identified as off-season, precompetition, competition, and transition. The delivery of training will then be on a microcycle basis involving planned training over small training periods, most often a week long. Each mesocycle will have specific training goals:

- *Off-season*: The emphasis at this stage is on preparation. Training volume and intensity build through this period, which is often seen as the hardest part of the training year. It lays the foundations for the competition period, and athletes will often work on those elements of their performance that are seen as weaknesses.
- *Precompetition*: The emphasis at this stage is on putting the finishing touches on the preparation period. In general, training at this point is sport-specific, with a greater emphasis on skills, speed, and power.
- *Competition*: The aims during this period depend upon the length of the competition season, but generally involve the maintenance of fitness built up in previous phases and the optimization of competition performance. Quality, rather than quantity, of training is emphasized, with sport-specific training dominating. In long seasons, this phase involves a delicate balance among training, competitions, and recovery.
- *Transition*: This stage is a crucial part of any program and involves active recovery from the season. Training intensity and volume are low, with an emphasis placed on recovery and regeneration from the effects of the season on a physical, psychological, and emotional level.

Prioritize and assign appropriate training loads.

It is impossible to work on all aspects of fitness at the same time. Therefore, it is vital to prioritize which aspects need to be the focus at any one time. This planning is intricately linked to the periodized plan outlined in the previous section. For example, a sprinter may develop his basic strength and speed endurance in the off-season and focus more on speed and power during the competition period.

It is important to identify areas of fitness that need to be developed, as well as those that need to be maintained at any given time. Doing so will influence the required training dose and the allocation of stimulating or maintenance loads. A maximum of three fitness parameters should be emphasized at a time, with the remaining parameters needed for the sport assigned as maintenance and given maintenance loads. Having prioritized which aspects of fitness are to be developed, the weekly training dose can be assigned.

Use the hard-easy principle.

It is impossible, and ill-advised, to take the body to the limit at all times, as doing so will almost undoubtedly lead to underrecovery and reduced levels of performance. When a fitness parameter is worked hard in one session, the intensity should be slightly lowered in the subsequent session. This pattern facilitates better recovery and ultimately better long-term gains.

Schedule recovery and regeneration.

Recovery and regeneration should be scheduled on a daily, weekly, monthly, and yearly basis. These schedules need to be as carefully planned as the training program itself, as it is the balance between the two that will ultimately bring about the best performance.

Physical Regeneration

Physical regeneration needs to become a part of every athlete's everyday life, and athletes should develop a number of tools to facilitate this element. Recovery should be proactive and in response to the training loads imposed. In this way, athletes learn to anticipate when they need to increase their recovery activities and make the necessary adjustments. Doing so can often prevent underrecovery.

Value inactivity.

For a self-disciplined athlete who is "making every minute count toward his goals," the value of periods of light activity or inactivity is often lost. Again, it is important to reiterate that training hard day-in and day-out for an extended period without adequate regeneration will reduce, not enhance, performance. Any effective training schedule will undulate training stresses to allow for recovery. This undulation will involve days of light activity and even days of inactivity. When these days are scheduled, it is vital that the athletes stick to them. They must be educated into eradicating the belief that training harder at these times will give better results. If athletes don't recover, they can't perform, and so they need to learn to value the regenerative-based activities as a vital part of their Performance Lifestyle.

Schedule light regeneration sessions.

Recovery needs to be proactive, and research has consistently shown that active recovery after training sessions results in better recovery than passive rest. In any training week, at least one session, and normally more, should be devoted to active recovery. Additionally, passive techniques can be used to supplement active techniques.

Relate recovery to the type and level of engagement.

The duration and frequency of regeneration activities needs to be related to the amount of training stress. By developing self-awareness, athletes should be able to identify times when they need to increase the number of recovery sessions undertaken. Recovery can thereby be enhanced, and the negative performance consequences of underrecovery can be minimized. Additionally, athletes will become aware of the type of fatigue associated with their type of training. They therefore can select methods of regeneration that best target the specific type of fatigue being experienced (refer to Figure 8-1).

Types of Regeneration Techniques

While a large number of strategies exist that can promote recovery, they can be classified into two types:

- Active regeneration techniques
- Passive regeneration techniques

ACTIVE REGENERATION TECHNIQUES

Active recovery sessions normally involve light activity and stretching. The intensity of these sessions must always be low (with a heart rate of less than 60 percent of maximum). Activities can vary among running, water-based activities, light cycling activities, playing other sports, etc. It is important that athletes develop a number of options for recovery sessions that they like and that promote recovery. At all times, it must be remembered that these sessions are recovery-based and must therefore be low intensity. Competition must never be allowed into these activities, as, given the competitive nature of athletes, work intensities will become too high and recovery will be compromised rather than enhanced. Active-recovery methods tend to work predominantly on the physiological level, and so need to be stressed at times when physiological fatigue is high. Additionally, many of the techniques can also promote psychological and emotional recovery.

Active regeneration should be performed on a daily basis. The preferred type of recovery activity, together with the quantity required, will depend upon the type and level of training stress and the aim of the training schedule. A number of strategies are available, all of which can be adapted to the specific needs of each athlete. The most basic and common active-recovery strategy is the cool-down, which can be performed after all training sessions and games. Additionally, other active-regeneration techniques exist that can contribute to recovery. It is important to remember that the effects of different strategies will be highly individualized, and that athletes need to develop their own recovery rituals to achieve optimal application. These rituals may simply involve the use of passive options such as ice baths or contrast showers, or may involve dedicated active-recovery sessions such as a pool session. Active regeneration techniques include the following: cool down/recovery routine, cross-training activities, and pool recovery session.

The Cool-Down/Recovery Routine

When to Use:

- As a cool-down session: Shortly after games, etc.; immediately following refuelling
- As a recovery session: At the end of the training day or in the morning of the subsequent day

Protocol: When used as a cool-down, the activities are preceded by a period of light activity for 2 to 10 minutes. The length of this activity is dependent upon the type of training undertaken. In general, the greater the physiological fatigue, the greater the length of preactivity. When used as a recovery session, it should be preceded by 5 to 10 minutes of light activity, such as jumping rope, light agility movements, etc.

Sample Session:

Kneeling Position (Figure 8-2)

- The athlete assumes a kneeling position with his knees hip-width apart.
- The tops of the feet and toes are flat on the floor, with the toes facing away.
- The athlete tucks in the tailbone and keeps his back flat.
- The body weight is back on the heels.
- The athlete reaches up and away with his arms, feeling a stretch through the upper body.

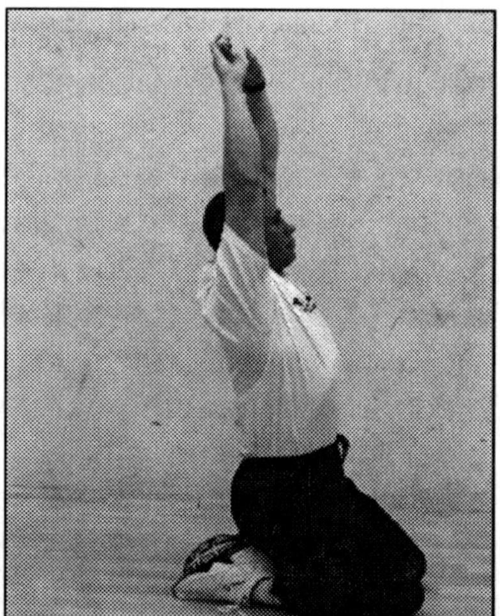

Figure 8-2

Camel (Figure 8-3)

- From the kneeling position, the athlete lifts the thighs upward and forward to a position perpendicular to the floor.

- The athlete tucks in the tailbone.
- At the same time, he arches the upper body backward.
- He the pulls the scapulae down and attempts to reach back and push the arms to the floor.
- With high levels of flexibility, the hands will be able to cup the ankles.

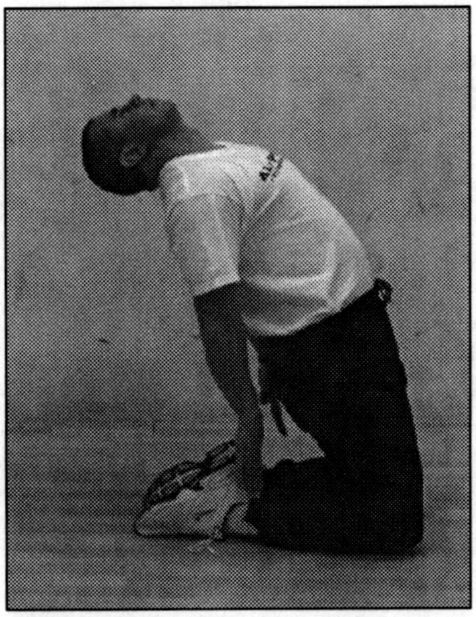

Figure 8-3

Child's Pose 1 (Figure 8-4)

- From the kneeling position, the athlete reaches his arms out in front.
- He then brings the forehead down toward the floor.
- He simultaneously pushes the arms away.
- The athlete should relax and feel the stretch through the upper body.

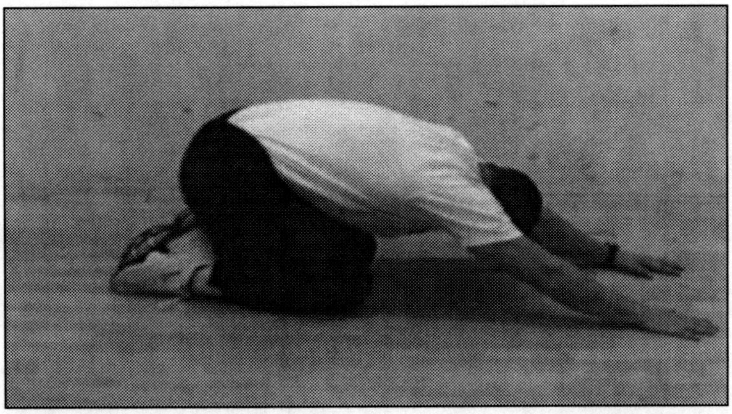

Figure 8-4

The Pike (Figure 8-5)

- The athlete begins in child's pose 1, with his arms pushed away and palms flat on the floor.
- He curls the toes under and presses the tailbone upward into an inverted V.
- The athlete then pushes the heels toward the floor.
- He squeezes his elbows together to roll the scapulae down and out.

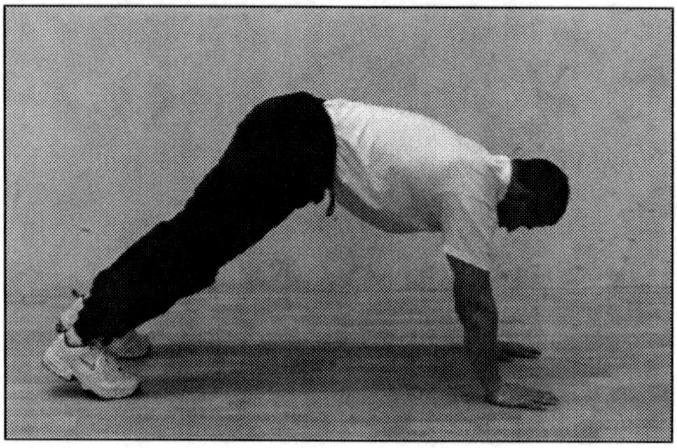

Figure 8-5

Upward-Facing Dog (Figure 8-6)

- From the pike position, the athlete brings the hips down to the ground.
- He places the tops of the feet flat on the floor.
- The athlete then pushes the hands into the floor, scooping the chest and abdominals up.
- The thighs can remain on the floor or slightly raised.
- The athlete pulls the scapulae down, pushing the chest forward.
- The athlete should try to achieve a straight line between the shoulders, elbows, and wrists.

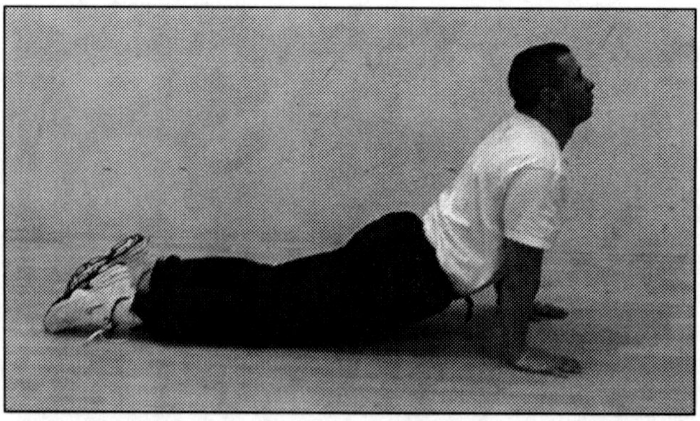

Figure 8-6

Child's Pose 2 (Figure 8-7)

- From upward-facing dog, the athlete resumes the kneeling position, but with his feet together and knees pushed out to 45 degrees.
- He reaches forward with the arms.
- He then brings the forehead toward the ground.

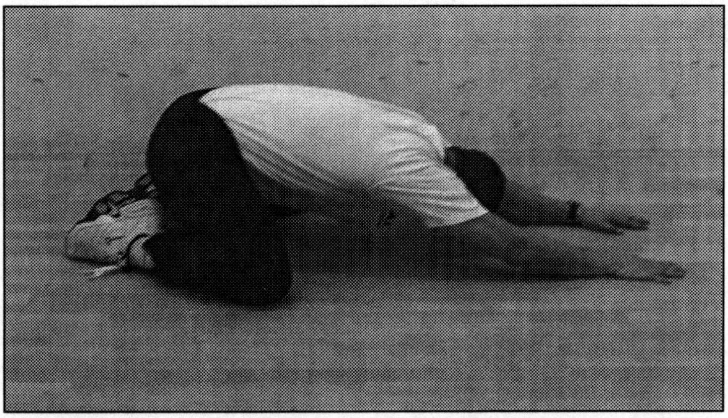

Figure 8-7

Frog (Figure 8-8)

- From child's pose 2, the athlete brings the knees out as far as possible.
- He rotates the feet to face out and bring his shins parallel to the knees.
- The thighs and shins should be at right angles.
- The athlete places the forearms flat on the floor, with the shoulders and elbows aligned.
- He raises the upper body and rests it on the forearms.
- He then lowers the hips back and down, pushing the knees out to the side.

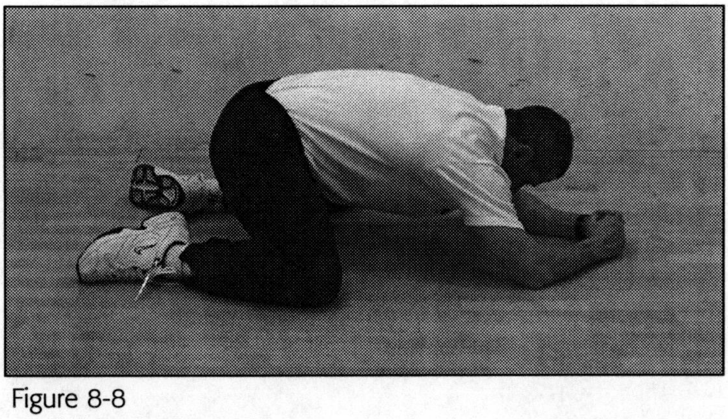

Figure 8-8

The Pike (Figure 8-9)

- From the frog position, the athlete narrows the knees and assumes the start position for the downward-facing dog.
- He curls the toes under and presses the tailbone upward into an inverted V.
- He pushes the heels toward the floor.
- He the squeezes his elbows together to roll the scapulae down and out.

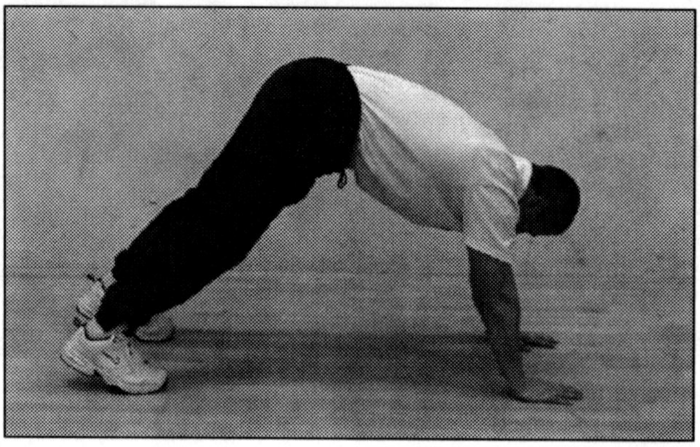

Figure 8-9

Warrior 1 (Figure 8-10)

- From the pike position, the athlete lunges the right foot forward between the hands.
- He then rotates the back foot to 90 degrees and assumes a long stance.
- He lowers the front leg to 90 degrees.
- He reaches the arms up and pushes away, simultaneously pushing the chest forward and up.
- The lower body should not rise.

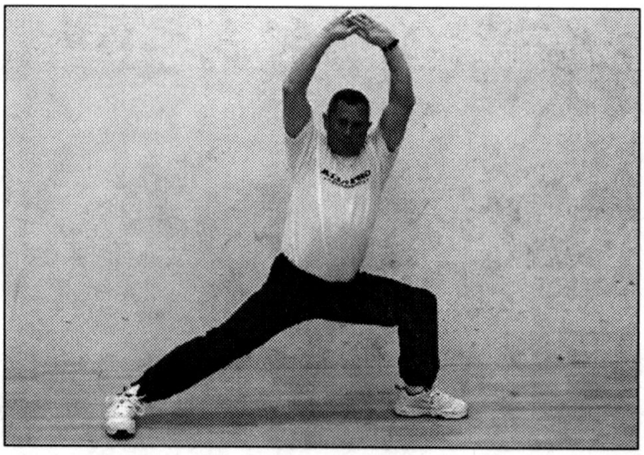

Figure 8-10

Extended Side Angle (Figure 8-11)

- From warrior 1, the athlete takes the opposite hand and places it flat on the floor.
- He raises the right arm straight up, creating a reaching feeling.
- He keeps the tailbone tucked under and the chest forward.

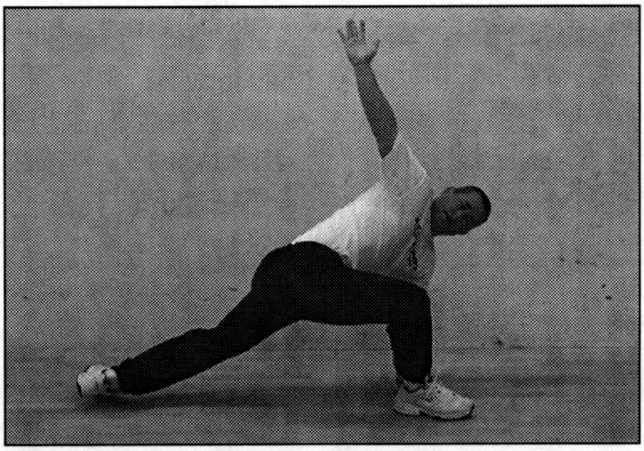

Figure 8-11

Warrior 2 (Figure 8-12)

- The athlete assumes the same position as for warrior 1.
- He rotates the body so that the front arm is pointing straight along the front leg.
- The chest should be square, with the scapulae pulled down.
- The athlete pushes the arms away in opposite directions.
- The warrior sequence should be repeated with a left foot lead.

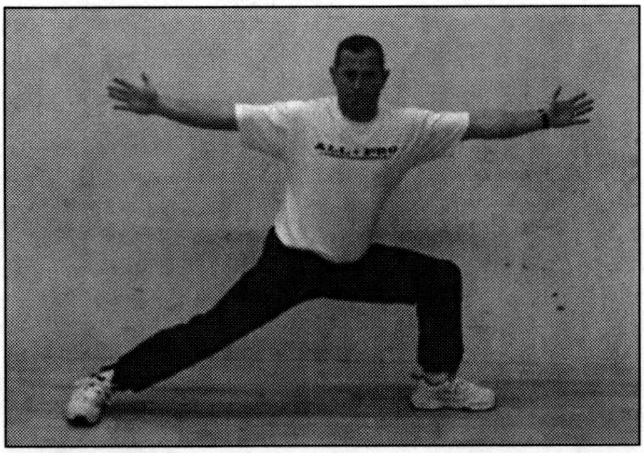

Figure 8-12

Lunge Sequence

- The athlete assumes a lunge position with the right leg forward and both feet facing forward.
- The body should be upright with the scapulae down and the chest forward and up.
- The athlete pushes the arms away (Figure 8-13).
- After 15 seconds, he leans the body in the direction of the forward leg, but with no forward or backward lean (Figure 8-14).
- After 15 seconds, he brings the upper body forward.
- He then places the left hand parallel to the right leg and rotates the body. He should hold this position for 15 seconds (Figure 8-15).
- The athlete should repeat the exercise, leading with the left side.

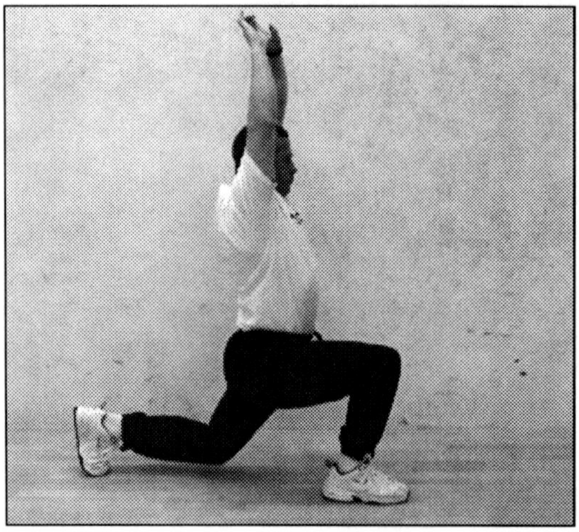

Figure 8-13

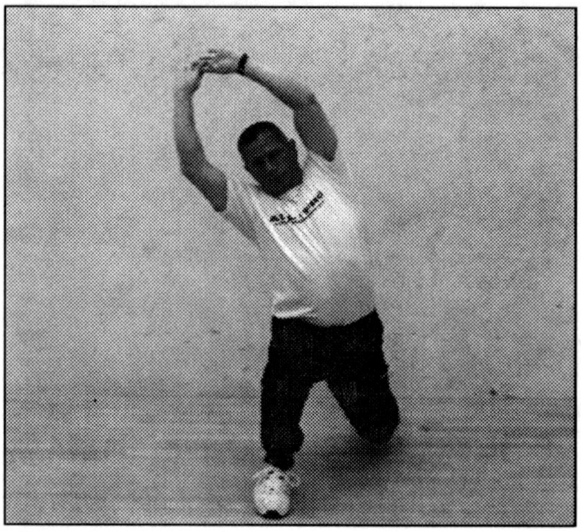

Figure 8-14

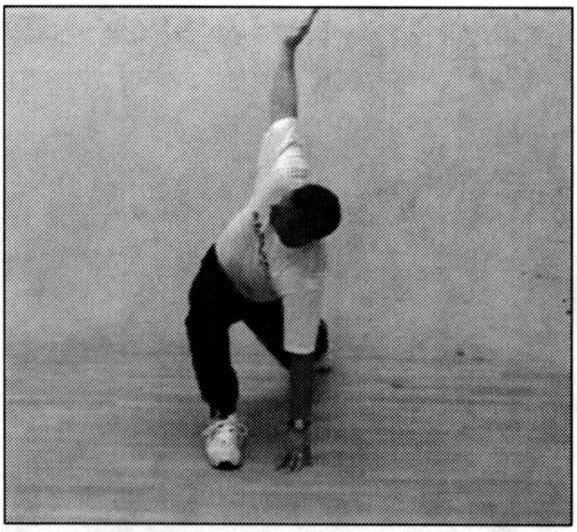

Figure 8-15

Squat (Figure 8-16)

- From the lunge position, the athlete assumes a full squat position.
- The feet should be hip-width apart, with the feet pointed ahead or slightly out and the heels flat.
- The athlete should aim to keep the upper body as upright as possible.
- He raises his arms overhead, pushing them backward.

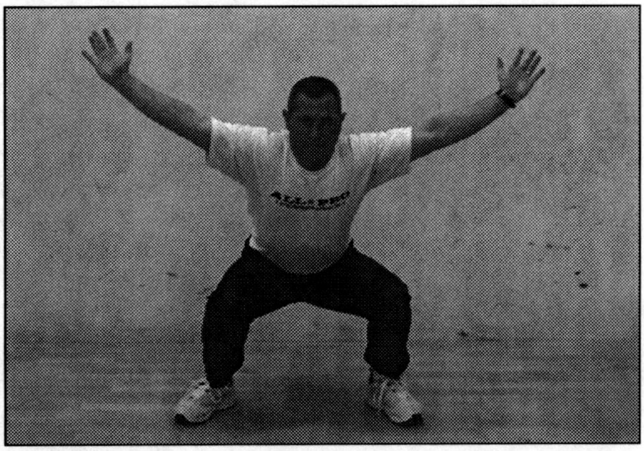

Figure 8-16

Single-Leg Reach (Figure 8-17)

- From the squat position, the athlete drops into a seated position with one leg forward and the other tucked into the thigh.
- Hinging at the hip, he reaches the chest forward toward the knee.
- The athlete should repeat this exercise, leading with the other leg.

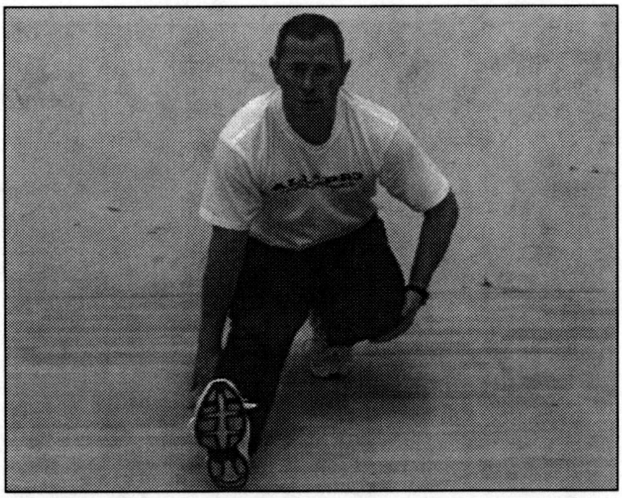

Figure 8-17

Double-Leg Reach (Figure 8-18)

- The athlete assumes a position similar to the single-leg reach, but with both legs extended.
- Hinging at the hip, he reaches the chest toward the knees.

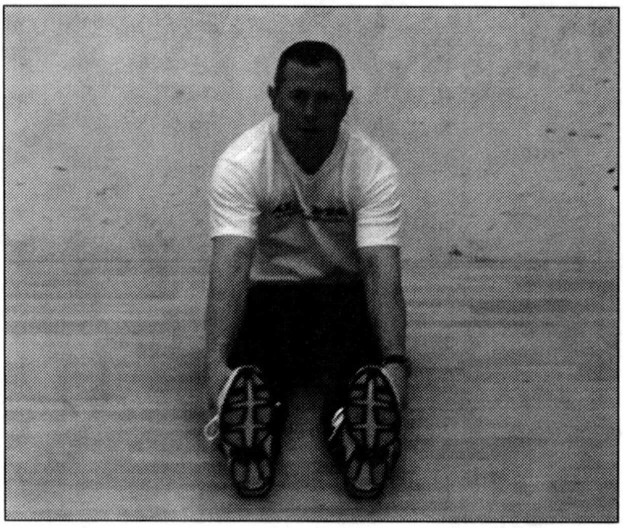

Figure 8-18

Tabletop (Figure 8-19)

- From the double-leg reach seated position, the athlete brings the hands back about a foot behind the hips with the palms flat and the fingers facing forward.
- He pushes into the floor and raises the hips.
- He then drops the head back.

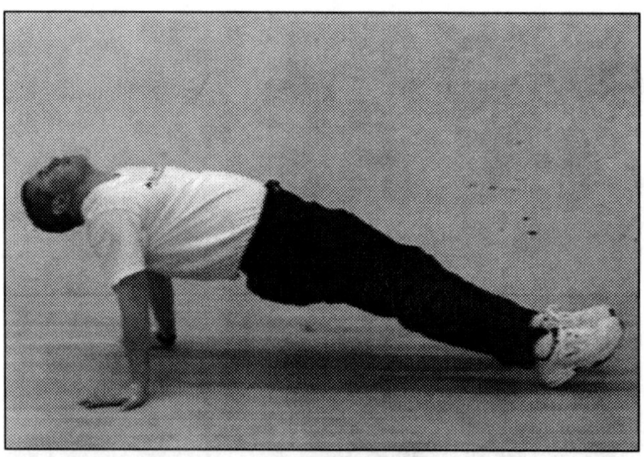

Figure 8-19

Supine Twist (Figure 8-20)

- From the tabletop position, the athlete returns to a seated position and then assumes a supine position with his arms in a crucifix position.
- He bends the right leg to 90 degrees and grabs the knee with the left hand.
- Keeping the right arm on the ground, he uses the left hand to pull the right knee toward the floor on the left side of his body.
- He then reverses the movement.

Reach (Figure 8-21)

- This exercise completes the routine and aims to elongate the spine.
- The athlete stands with his feet together and tucks the tailbone in.
- He reaches to the sky with his arms straight and palms together.
- He tilts the head back, looking to the sky.
- He attempts to push down with the feet and up with the arms.

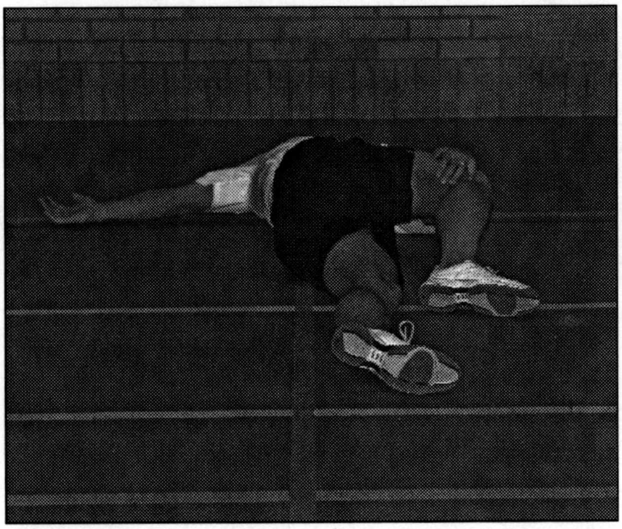

Figure 8-20

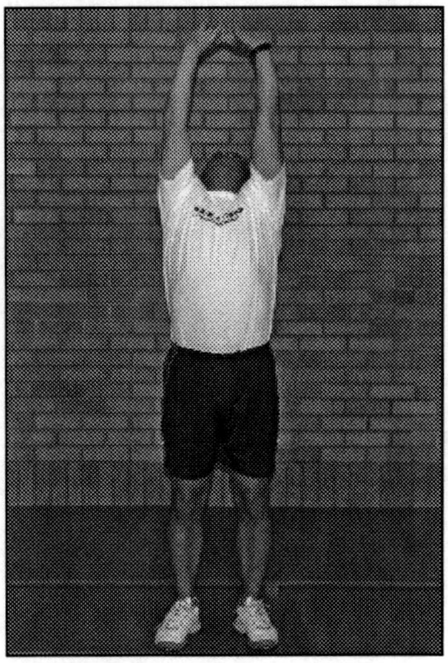

Figure 8-21

Cross-Training Activities

Participating in other activities can provide recovery on a psychological, emotion, and physical level. Athletes should choose activities that they enjoy, and which can be performed at a low intensity. Heavy athletes may also consider choosing activities that provide low-impact loads, such as swimming.

When to Use: These exercises should be incorporated into the training program on a macro-, meso-, and microcycle basis.

Protocol: Whatever activity is chosen, it must be performed at a low intensity. The aim is recovery. Therefore, activities should not lead to additional fatigue.

Sample Session: The athlete can perform a very gentle cycle ride for 20 to 30 minutes.

Pool Recovery Session

Pool recovery sessions provide a suitable tool with which to facilitate physiological and neural recovery. An advantage of this method is that the water provides for an environment in which both activation and mobilization can take place without a large degree of impact.

When to Use: At the end of the training day, or first thing in the morning after a strenuous game or training session

Protocol: Pool workouts normally start with activities that raise the heart rate and metabolism, followed by activities that mobilize the major joints. Work intensity should be low at all times. Remember, the aim is to recover, not to expend energy. If an athlete is not a great swimmer, and swimming uses up energy, he should take a greater break between the swimming actions or walk at intervals during the swim. When swimming strokes are used, the aim is to use full range of motion to allow for appropriate mobilization.

Sample Session (assuming a 25-meter pool):

The athletes:

- Swim three lengths, alternating backstroke, breaststroke, and front crawl
- Walk for three minutes in waist-high water using a range of upper-body activities (e.g., sprint action, reaching up, side bends, rotations)
- Walk two widths using full high-knee action in shoulder-high water
- Walk two faster widths using high-knee running action in shoulder-high water
- Walk two widths with an ankling action in waist-high water
- Swim two lengths, sidestroke (alternate sides)
- Walk two widths sideways using a side-lunge action in waist-high water
- Swim three lengths, alternating backstroke, front crawl, and backstroke
- Walk two widths using crossover steps in waist-high water
- Walk two widths with a hip circling action in shoulder-high water (width 1 forward, width 2 backward)
- Walk two widths, lunging in waist-high water with a variety of lunging combinations
- Walk two widths backward, taking large steps in waist-high water.

- Swim two lengths sidestroke (alternating sides)
- Walk two widths with a sprinter's paw-back action in waist-high water.
- Walk two widths with a high kick action in waist-high water
- Jog two widths in waist-high water
- Spend five minutes statically stretching key muscles in the water

PASSIVE REGENERATION TECHNIQUES

In addition to active recovery sessions, passive methods can be used to further enhance recovery. Passive techniques include hydrotherapy, contrast showers, and self-massage. These methods are especially useful when neural fatigue is predominant and when the need for physiological recovery is less pronounced. Again, a range of rituals needs to be developed that can be utilized in all locations and at all times. Passive recovery options include the following techniques: self-massage, contrast showers, ice baths, contrast bathing, compression clothing.

Self-Massage

Massage is a valuable tool in an athlete's recovery arsenal. Whenever possible, an athlete should use a qualified therapist who will be able to manipulate the type of massage to his requirements. However, it is not always possible to do so, and the following self-massage technique is a great alternative.

When to Use: This technique can be used at any time, but is more effective post-workout or at the end of the day.

Protocol: The self-massage protocol requires three pieces of equipment. The major one is a foam roller, which is extremely useful. The athlete leans his body against the roller, with the movement of the body providing the massage. Additionally, a massage stick can be used to access areas that require additional work, such as the calves. Tennis balls are used in a similar way to massage small points that need greater attention.

Athletes should massage each area for as long as they feel it is giving benefit. The length of the session will therefore depend upon the need for massage, which will be related to the work performed that day.

Sample Session: The athlete should massage the following areas, using the equipment noted:

- Calves—stick (Figure 8-22)
- Hamstrings—foam roller (Figure 8-23)
- Iliotibial band (which runs down the outside of the leg)—foam roller (Figure 8-24)

- Quadriceps—foam roller (Figure 8-25)
- Inner thighs—foam roller (Figure 8-26)
- Lower back—foam roller (Figure 8-27)
- Upper back—foam roller (Figure 8-28)
- Glutes—foam roller (Figure 8-29)
- Lats—foam roller (Figure 8-30)
- Feet—tennis ball (Figure 8-31)

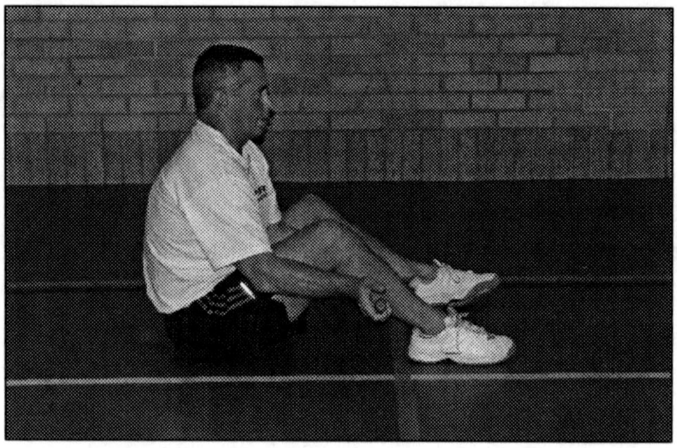

Figure 8-22

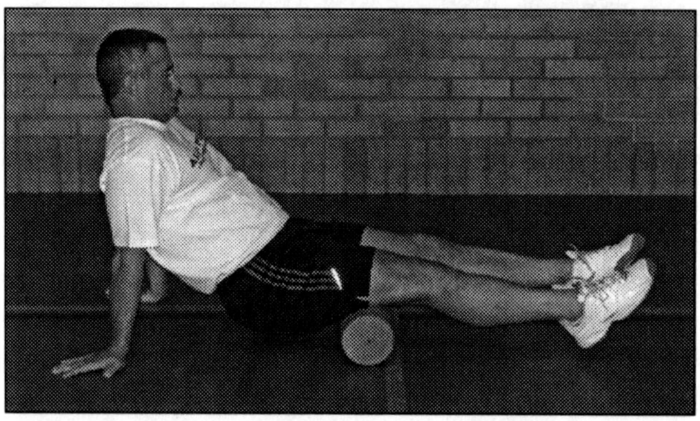

Figure 8-23

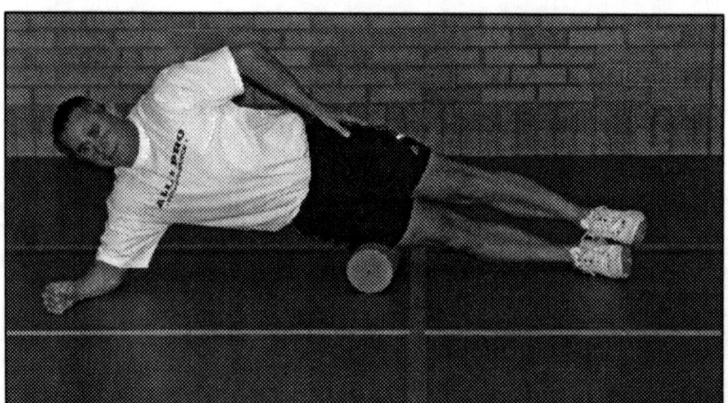

Figure 8-24

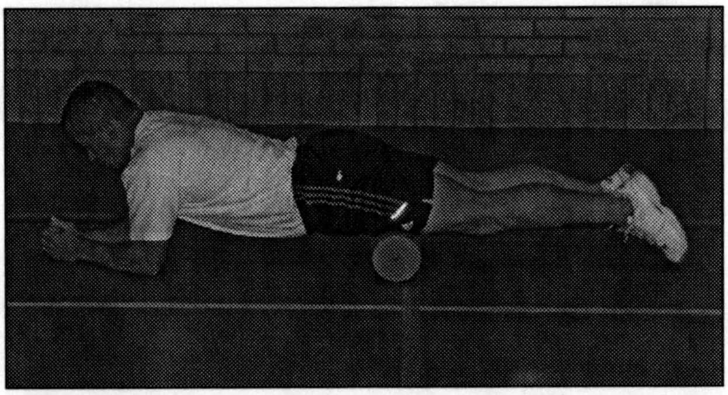
Figure 8-25

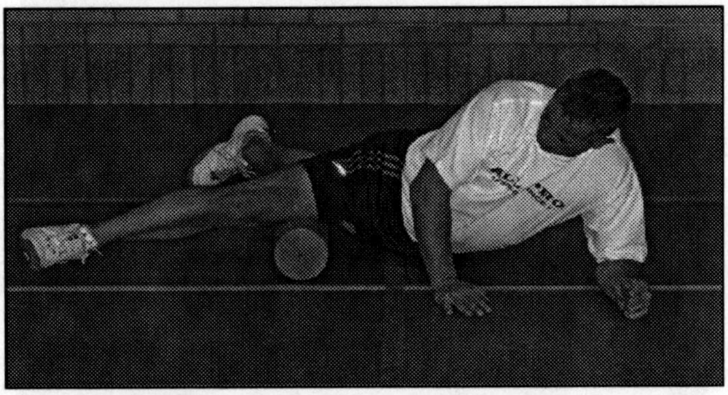
Figure 8-26

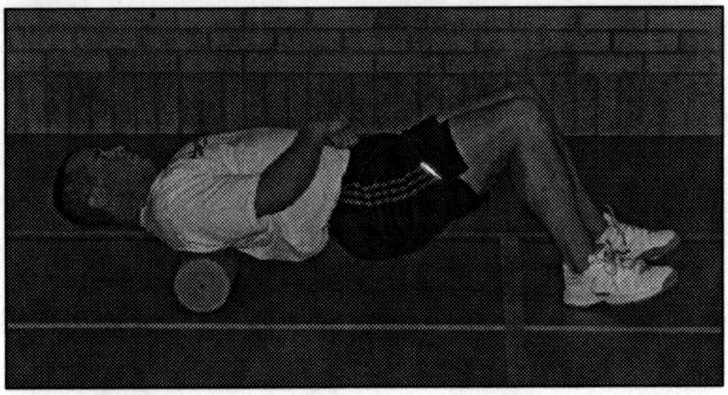
Figure 8-27

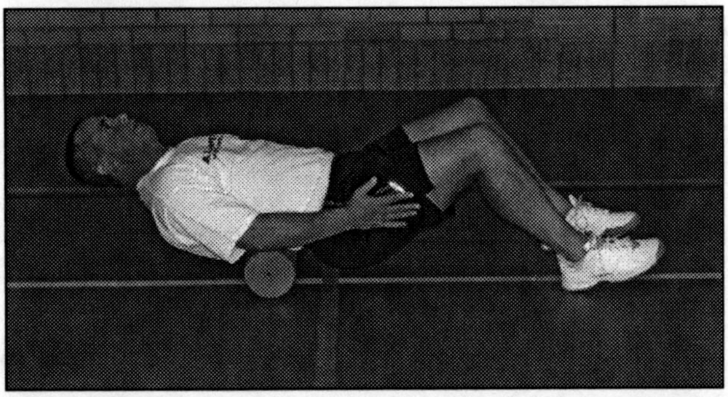
Figure 8-28

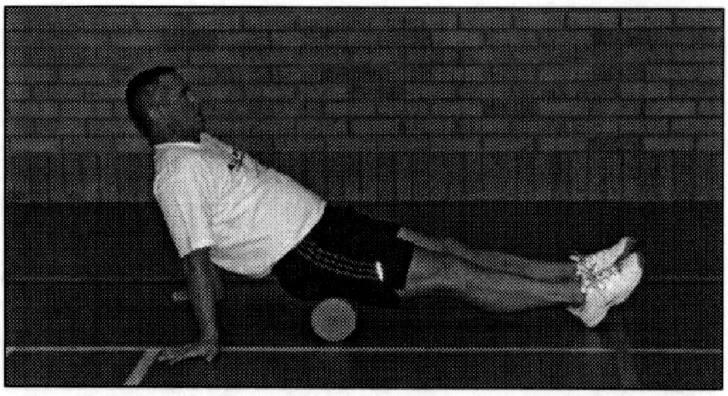

Figure 8-29

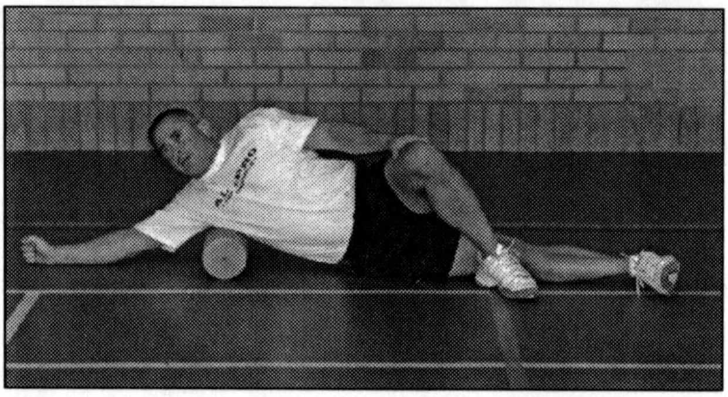

Figure 8-30

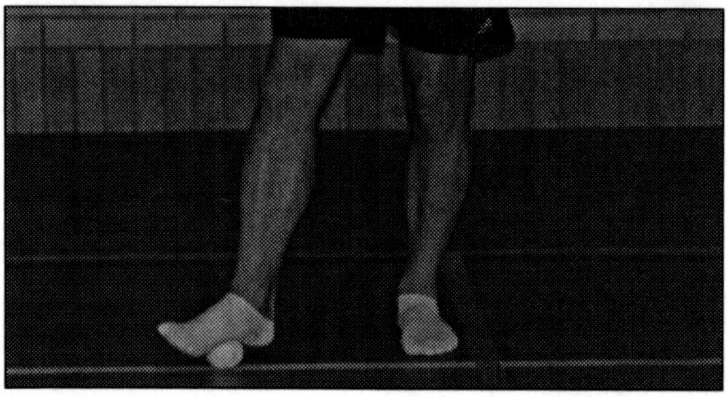

Figure 8-31

Contrast Showers

Alternating between cold and warm showers facilitates neural recovery and provides for a psychological pick-up.

When to Use: Contrast showers can be used at any time, especially where rapid recovery is required.

Protocol: The athlete should use water that is as cold as bearable and as hot as bearable. Doing so provides for a greater degree of contrast.

Sample Session: The athlete alternates 30 seconds of cold with one minute of hot, and repeats three times. He should finish with the hot shower.

Ice Baths

Ice baths are a suitable postmatch recovery tool and end-of-day activity.

When to Use: Ice baths can be used immediately after games/training or at the end of the day.

Protocol: The athlete should use water that is as cold as bearable and submerge the main areas of the body for the allotted time. In many cases, it is the lower body that requires the submersion.

Sample Session: The athlete submerges the body in cold water for two minutes, followed by a normal warm shower.

Contrast Bathing

Alternating between cold and warm baths facilitates both physiological and neural recovery. Additionally, when hot tubs can be used to provide the warm immersion, the use of warm jets can provide massage to areas in need of additional attention.

When to Use: Contrast bathing should be used at the end of the training day.

Protocol: The athlete should use water that is as cold as bearable and as hot as bearable. Doing so provides for a greater degree of contrast. This method should not be used if athletes are suffering from a soft-tissue injury.

Sample Session: The athlete should alternate 30 seconds of cold immersion with two minutes of hot immersion, repeated three times. If possible, he should use the jets to massage areas that need additional attention, such as the calves or hamstrings. He should finish with the hot bath.

Compression Clothing

Garments that provide compression may provide a useful tool in facilitating recovery.

When to Use: Compression clothing can be worn immediately following training and through the night.

Protocol: Compression garments should be worn following the cool-down and any other recovery activities. They can be worn through the night for additional benefit.

Why Passive Regeneration Techniques Work

All of the passive regeneration methods just described are based on their capacity to increase or decrease the level of activation of the cortex and subcortical systems of the brain, and their involvement in the overall processes of central nervous system regulation. They also work to increase venous and muscle blood flow, facilitating recovery by removing metabolites and delivering the required building blocks of recovery.

Optimizing Regeneration Results

When to Use Recovery Tools

The best time to use the recovery tools depends upon recovery requirements. If recovery needs to be immediate (e.g., between morning and afternoon workouts), the best time to use them is immediately after training. In these instances, short-term tools such as contrast showers and self-massage are the best options. When the aim is to recover over a longer time period (e.g., before the next day's training), it is better to use the strategies six to nine hours after training. These techniques will take the form of long-term strategies. When competition or training ends in the evening, the next day is the best time to deploy the strategies:

- *Short-term strategies*: Contrast showers and localized massage
- *Long-term strategies*: Pool workouts, ice baths, contrast bathing, full-body massage

Local or General Strategies

Whether it is best to use localized or full-body strategies depends upon the type of fatigue experienced. Full-body strategies, such as contrast showers, are best used after large volumes of general training. Local methods, such as massage, are best used when work that strongly stresses specific muscle groups is performed.

Tool Variation

As with training, the overall effectiveness of any physical-restoration tool will vary over time. No tool is universally better than any other, and the effectiveness will vary among individuals and at different times. The key is to vary the applications, using different strategies at different times to optimize the results. Each athlete should try a number of strategies and evaluate how they work for him, and then integrate them into his program. It should also be noted that the strategies have the capacity to work on different levels, which can help athletes select appropriate strategies. Therefore, if an athlete finds that he dislikes one strategy, and that the thought of it creates psychological stress, he can replace it with one he does like and that works for him.

THE PSYCHOLOGICAL DOMAIN

Psychological performance contributes massively to the overall performance levels of athletes, and to their capacity to regenerate and recover. As with the physical domain, it is important that the psychological capacity is developed via appropriate strategies, together with the use of effective psychological regeneration strategies, to optimize recovery.

Developing Psychological Capacity

Psychological skills are vital tools in the arsenal of any athlete, both to optimize performance and facilitate recovery. By building psychological capacity, athletes are better able to cope with the psychological pressures of the performance environment and everyday life.

The development of psychological skills is a huge topic that is beyond the scope of this book. However, just like a physical-training program, psychological training needs to be geared to developing the individual's specific needs. A starting point is the psychological-skills profile outlined in the self-awareness pillar (refer to Chapter 5), which identifies the key target areas that will bring the most benefit to the athlete, and that need to be the focus of the program. Areas of weakness need to be targeted, with the athlete aiming to climb the wall toward developing a higher level of psychological performance. Climbing the wall is the process of constantly aiming to enhance psychological capacity. It is key that the athlete identifies the psychological areas that are affecting his performance. The psychological profile carried out in Pillar 2 (refer to Chapter 5) is an ideal starting point, as are the Performance Reviews outlined later in the book. Using these methods, key target areas can be identified, and the athlete's capacity in each of these areas can be enhanced.

Again, this text is insufficient to cover the whole gamut of psychological training techniques, and athletes should consult with a sport psychologist and follow a well-designed program. What is important is that psychological training becomes part of daily and weekly rituals, which will enhance performance and provide the techniques to ensure optimal recovery.

Psychological Regeneration

Just as it is impossible to sustain high training intensities or volumes for extended periods, it is impossible to sustain high psychological outputs such as intense concentration, focusing, analyzing, and learning for extended periods of time. While these skills are developed via the capacity-building process, it is important that the athlete can have periods during which these requirements are switched off, and when athletes can experience periods of calmness, relaxation, creativity, and decreased focus, which are the characteristics of the psychological regeneration states that the Performance Lifestyle encourages.

As outlined in Pillar 3 (refer to Chapter 6), to experience effective recovery and regeneration, athletes want to be in the positive, low-energy portion of the quadrant. To achieve this state and feel relaxed, content, etc., they need to be psychologically disengaged. While this guideline may seem straightforward, athletes will often ruminate over performances, thereby producing a stream of negative thoughts, especially if they have experienced failure.

Long-Term Versus Short-Term Recovery

The psychological domain has a massive effect on recovery. In many instances, the perception of stress and fatigue may be more powerful than the stress itself. By altering perceptions and thoughts, athletes are often better able to manage the stressor and stay in the positive quadrant. The ABCD exercise outlined in Chapter 6 is a key way in which athletes can alter their beliefs and thoughts. While these processes take place over the long term, a need to psychologically recover in the short term also exists, based on how well athletes are able to disengage from any matter that is causing stress.

Rumination—A Key Cause of Psychological Stress

Rumination refers to the process whereby an event is replayed constantly in the mind. It normally involves negative questioning about the event, such as "What if I had done something differently?" While the ABCD and inner-voice activities carried out in Pillar 3 (refer to Chapter 6) will hopefully have reduced any pessimistic trends and developed an overall level of optimism, athletes will still experience negative thoughts every now and again. This process is natural and should not in itself be an undue cause for concern. Indeed, being aware of negative emotions is a key part of the self-awareness pillar (refer to Chapter 5). What is vital, though, is that athletes do not ruminate. Negative thoughts going round and round in their heads are unlikely ever to be of benefit, and will undoubtedly sap their energy.

When negative emotions are evident, athletes must take note of them, but then be able to disengage. Unfortunately, thoughts can pop up in an athlete at the most inopportune time, and problems are often caused by thoughts that are either inappropriately timed or inappropriately targeted. For example, as a player prepares for a key penalty shot in soccer, focusing on the consequences of missing (e.g., his friends ridiculing him, letting the team down) is not the best strategy. In these instances, the athlete needs to ask, "Is this the best thing to be thinking about right now?" In most cases, it certainly is not. Instead, the focus should be on the action of taking the penalty shot. Athletes need to be able to develop the ability to put problems off to another time—a process called active disengagement.

Active Disengagement

An athlete's ability to take his mind off the issues facing him is a vital disengagement tool. Everyone has lied in bed unable to sleep because of the worries and issues racing through their mind. Whatever the cause of these thoughts, the simple truth is that the issue is not going to be resolved or go away as the person lies there. In fact, losing sleep will likely decrease the chances of effectively tackling the issue. In many instances, the reality of the problem the next day is seldom the issue a person sees it as during the night. By actively disengaging, athletes can reduce the stress and agree to tackle the problem at a more appropriate time.

The strategy outlined in Figure 8-32 can be used to help disengage from the problem for a period of time. This strategy involves identifying and acknowledging that the issue exists, not ignoring it. Indeed, issues should never be ignored, as they provide the potential to become major energy sappers. Instead, the process acknowledges the problem, but sets aside a time and place when it is appropriate to address it. In this way, the problem is set aside for a time (the recovery time), and addressed at a later, more opportune time.

Disengagement

What is bothering you?

What problems is this issue causing?

When are you going to deal with this problem?

What are you going to do?

Figure 8-32

It is important that the athlete comes back to these issues at the agreed upon time. Otherwise, his subconscious mind will never trust itself and will not disengage the next time. Again, coming back to the problem needs to be a ritual. Figure 8-33 shows how the disengagement strategy can be deployed for an athlete worried about a coach's criticism.

Disengagement

What is bothering you?

Coach was really down on me today. Perhaps he's going to drop me for the next game. Every mistake I made, he picked up on it and made it a point in front of the whole team.

What problems is this issue causing?

This issue is making me feel really miserable. I can't think of anything else and I'm not even enjoying being with my friends. Thinking like this will mean that I can't concentrate on my schoolwork and probably means that I won't sleep tonight.

When are you going to deal with this problem?

Tomorrow at practice

What are you going to do?

I'm going to ask Coach for a talk, to see how he thinks I'm doing and what I need to do to get better. Then I'm going to spend 10 minutes each session working on the things that he thinks I need to work on.

Figure 8-33

The very act of writing a problem down is a great disengagement strategy. When a problem is written down, its severity is often very much reduced. In many instances, the perceived problems are greater than the reality and the negative emotions disappear without the need for deeper analysis. This fact stresses the vital role of the general comments in the daily training/recovery log in the disengagement process, and subsequently the recovery process. However, if the negative thoughts reoccur, they might be a warning of deeper issues and need to be addressed via the ABCD system outlined in Pillar 3 (refer to Chapter 6).

While the best approach to the problem is to write it down—what gets measured gets done—it is not always possible to do so. In these instances, the same approach can be used, but utilizing the mind rather than paper. The athlete again identifies the thoughts and agrees to deal with them later, but this information is logged in the mind rather than on paper. Again, it is important that the athlete commits to this process later.

Relaxation Techniques

Relaxation can bring about an ideal recovery state on a physical, psychological, and emotional basis. When possible, athletes need to include relaxation rituals within their day. These tools are especially useful prior to bedtime or after particularly stressful days. By relaxing, athletes are increasing the likelihood of reaching the positive, low-energy part of the quadrant, which is associated with optimal recovery. Relaxation can be achieved in a number of ways, but it is important that athletes are able to remain undisturbed for the period of time required.

A progressive relaxation system is outlined in the following section. Many of the activities used to enhance emotional regeneration will contribute to the positive, low-energy relaxed psychological states required for psychological regeneration.

Progressive Relaxation

Progressive relaxation is based upon experiencing the difference between tension and relaxation by progressively tensing and then relaxing different body parts until a feeling of total relaxation in achieved. This process is best practiced after a disengagement strategy is used to enable the mind to feel at rest and relaxed.

When to Use: This tool can be used any time an athlete needs to increase relaxation, but works best when sufficient time is available to allow for an uninterrupted session.

Protocol: The athlete lies on his back in a quiet, comfortable place, where he will not be disturbed. He should dim the lights and loosen any clothing. He then takes a deep breath and lets it out slowly. He should repeat this breath three more times.

With his arms lying to his sides, he clenches his fists as hard as possible for five seconds. He should feel the tension in the hands and fingers and then let go. He should compare the relaxation with the tension felt when the fists were clenched, and feel how the tension drains away when the fists are relaxed. He should feel the relaxation for 15 seconds.

Next, he tenses the upper arms for five seconds, feeling the tension. He lets this tension go and then feels the relaxation for 15 seconds, feeling the arms hang loosely by his sides.

Next he focuses on the toes, curling them as tightly as possible for five seconds, followed by 15 seconds of relaxation.

He then turns his attention to the following areas in sequence, repeating the pattern of five seconds of tension followed by 15 seconds of relaxation:

- Feet and calves (pointing the toes away)
- Thighs
- Stomach
- Chest and shoulders (pressing the palms together)
- Back (by squeezing the shoulder blades together)
- Neck (bringing the chin to the chest)

Once this cycle is done, he should focus on breathing deeply and rhythmically, breathing in for two seconds, holding in the chest for five seconds, and exhaling for 10 seconds. At the same time, he should feel relaxation in all of the body parts previously addressed. The athlete should take five minutes to experience this deep relaxation. He should remain in this relaxed position for as long as he feels the need. To optimize the experience, the mind should remain disengaged.

The Performance Review—A Key Disengagement Tool

Competition provides the most intense level of stress placed on an athlete. Stress is intense during the competition and can spill over for a considerable time after competition. When competition does not go well, the negative emotions generated can last for many days. A key strategy for reducing this level of postperformance stress is the performance review, which should be completed as soon as possible after a competition (Figure 8-34).

Athletes need to ensure that they highlight as many good points as possible and don't simply make it a total criticism of their performance, especially if the result did not go their way. They need to use positive, optimistic language and should finish by using the data to help them in the goal-setting process for the coming week. In this way, they can start to disengage from the performance and start the process of moving forward toward their goals. This process will also reduce their rumination time, which is a major cause of psychological stress. Figure 8-35 shows a completed analysis.

THE EMOTIONAL DOMAIN

As with the psychological domain, emotional aspects of performance are underdeveloped and can provide a massive increase in overall stress capacity. The emotionally healthy athlete has a large stress tolerance. However, the reverse is also

Performance Review

Opponents ______________________________________ Date ________________

Venue ________________________Competition _____________________________

General details of the game:

How did you feel coming into the game?

List those things you did well in this game (physical, psychological, technical, tactical).

List those things you could have done better in this game (physical, psychological, technical, tactical).

What can you learn from this game?

Figure 8-34

Performance Review

Opponents: United — Date: August 20, 2006

Venue: Home ground — Competition: League

General details of the game:

The first game of the season, played in high temperatures, with an early start

How did you feel coming into the game?

I felt nervous, as this was the first game and we didn't know how we would perform, but generally confident, as training had gone well. My fitness scores were at record levels, which gave me confidence. The early start time meant I had not eaten since breakfast

List those things you did well in this game (physical, psychological, technical, tactical).

Physically, I was strong throughout most of the game, and my speed was excellent. My technique was good, and I felt confident, despite them being a very good team. Tactically, I was able to carry out my role within the team.

List those things you could have done better in this game (physical, psychological, technical, tactical).

Focus on the performance and not the score during the game.
Take on more fluids during the game, starting right at the start.
Alter my eating patterns to reflect the start time.

What can you learn from this game?

Ensure adequate food and fluid intake before and during the game.
Have a performance focus rather than a score focus.

Figure 8-35

true, so when emotional health breaks down, performance in all areas comes tumbling down.

As with the other domains, emotional development requires the development of emotional capacity, together with the utilization of activities that can enhance emotional regeneration.

Developing Emotional Capacity

An athlete's emotional capacity is closely linked to his emotional intelligence. Emotional intelligence refers to ability in four key areas, which according to Daniel Goleman (1995), are:

- Self-awareness
- Self-control
- Social awareness
- Social control

As with all of the capacity-developing elements, emotional capacity will be developed by building the athlete's capacity in each of these four areas.

Developing Self-Awareness

The process of developing self-awareness will have started with the self-awareness tools used in developed in Pillar 2 (refer to Chapter 5). The ability to identify both positive and negative emotions needs to be cultivated. Once these emotions are identified, it is important to start to identify the causes of the emotions. When the causes of positive emotions can be identified, they can be used as a starting point to be able to recreate these emotions as required. The use of triggers can be used to help recreate positive states.

The use of triggers is simply an extension of the movies technique used in Pillar 1 (refer to Chapter 4). This tool is a process by which an athlete can attach a phrase or action to a particular image. For example, an athlete may associate a place he has visited to a feeling of tranquillity and contentment. By developing the image of that place through the use of the movies technique, a name can be attached to that movie. Whenever he uses that name or trigger, it has the capacity to make the athlete feel tranquil and content, which are both important low-energy, positive emotions. Over time, whenever he says the name of the place, he will bring up the image he has developed, which will assist him in developing a feeling of tranquillity and contentment, as and when needed. Similarly, other triggers can be developed to create other emotional feelings. Figure 8-36 outlines a method athletes can use to develop positive emotional triggers.

Developing Triggers

- Identify a positive emotion you wish to create.
- Picture a time when you felt this way.
- Look at the picture. Picture yourself in the middle of the movie, just as if you are watching yourself achieving your success. Now pay attention to the size of the image, making it as big as possible. Next look at the colors, and make them as vivid as possible. Next switch up the brightness, just as you would on a TV set. The aim is to make the picture as clear and vivid as possible. Watch this movie for a while.
- Next turn to the sound, or what you can hear. Again, play with the controls and make the sounds as loud and real as you can.
- Then turn to any smells, tastes, or feelings that you can imagine. These senses may not always be applicable, but remember that the more real the image, the better the result.
- Attach a trigger word to this image. Each time you picture the image reemphasize the trigger word.
- Over time, the use of this trigger will be able to recreate the emotion.

Figure 8-36

In addition to being aware of positive emotions, athletes also need to become aware of negative emotions. When negative emotions are identified, they need to be embraced, not suppressed. Negative emotions normally stem from stressful environments, and if ignored can result in high anxiety and arousal levels. These high levels can drain energy on a psychosocial level and result in underrecovery. When negative emotions are identified, they need to lead to a deeper analysis, as outlined in the ABCD activities in Pillar 2 (refer to Chapter 5). Once the cause of the negative emotion is identified, strategies and rituals can be used to attempt to reduce these causes.

Developing Self-Control

There is a gap between stimulus and response. During this time, athletes have the right and ability to make choices.

How many times have you reacted spontaneously to someone and said things that you later regretted? An athlete's ability to control what he says and does in these times is dependent upon his level of self-control. Self-control, in turn, is dependent largely upon self-awareness (e.g., an athlete can identify times that he is irritable, and, rather than react angrily to something that has annoyed him, recognize his irritability and choose to say nothing). Lack of self-control can often lead to unwanted outbursts both on and off the field of play, which simply increases stress levels.

Consider the following example: A cornerback has just been beaten on an outside route and, in his frustration, pushes the receiver when he is out of bounds and is called for unnecessary roughness. This penalty results in him experiencing the wrath of the coach, which in turn results in more frustration. Losing his focus on the next play, he tries to bump the receiver instead of playing him deep, and is subsequently beaten deep for the game-winning touchdown. During the next week, this sequence is the focus of many film and training sessions, and he feels responsible for the loss. During the week, he feels lethargic and drained of energy and is unable to relax. Had he shown self-control after the first mistake, then the whole sequence of events that followed the loss of control may have been avoided, and the stress levels for the whole week would have been very different. While extreme, this example does demonstrate how self-control can assist in reducing stress.

When faced with a stressful situation, athletes need to learn to hit the stop button. Before reacting, they need to think, "What do I want to achieve here, and what is the likely result if I respond in this way?" This pause can give athletes time to react in an appropriate manner and is vital in developing self-control. Another useful question is, "When I look back at this situation in a week or so, will I regret what I am about to do?" The creation of this thinking time between stimulus and response is crucial for developing self-control.

Developing Social Awareness

All relationships with others have great potential for recovery, but also have great potential for stress. All actions an athlete carries out can impact upon other people in some way or another. In many instances, these people will play an important role in athletes' lives—people such as coaches, teammates, friends, and parents. When these relationships are good, they can provide for an ideal recovery environment. However, where these relationships are strained, they can cause huge amounts of psychological and emotional stress.

The key strategy in developing effective social awareness is to see the other person's point of view and focus on how any actions will appear to him. Sometimes this viewpoint may be quite different from that of the athlete, but by attempting to see this point of view, the athletes are building a bridge to the other person. The athlete can still make his point, but he needs to do it in way that does not alienate the other person.

For example, a new team member is extremely shy and finds it difficult to engage with his new teammates. Instead, he chooses to keep quiet and just get on with his job. However, some teammates start to misconstrue this behavior as arrogance and start to talk with other teammates negatively about the shy athlete, using comments such as, "He thinks he's better than us." If this situation continues, it has the capacity to cause stress for the shy athlete, who may start to feel alienated from the team, which can further exacerbate the shyness. In the long term, the stress caused by this situation would be far greater than that caused by having to make an effort to communicate with his teammates in the first place. Developing the social awareness of the consequences of his actions would be a very important development for this athlete, together with the development of social skills to assist in communication.

Developing Social Control

The development of social control is the next step of social awareness and involves the development of skills to deal with potentially stressful situations. The socially skilled athlete is able to do so in a way that allows him to deal with an issue without alienating other people, and while maintaining his self-respect.

For example, a time may arise when an athlete is dropped from the team. While he may not agree with the decision, the coach is likely doing what he considers the best thing for the team at that point. Rather than argue or complain, the socially aware athlete will ask the coach why he's been dropped and, in a calm manner, ask for advice on how to improve his performance. In this way, a personal relationship can be maintained, or even enhanced, creating the potential for a stress-free environment. Social skills are especially important when dealing with the media, where mistakes are recorded, played back, and can cause extremely high levels of stress.

Emotional Disengagement

Emotional disengagement and subsequent recovery are vital for optimal health, and for optimal recovery. Emotional recovery will occur most effectively when the emotions associated with the positive, low-energy quarter of the energy quadrant are achieved. Worry, anger, sadness, frustration, etc., will all hinder recovery. Athletes need to be able to engage in activities that foster feelings such as contentment, relaxation, and enjoyment. To achieve this emotional regeneration, a number of key elements need to be addressed.

Ensure that emotional needs are addressed.

One of the biggest energy drains is unmet needs, whether on a physical, psychological, or emotional level. Unfulfilled needs equal stress. In pillar 1 (refer to Chapter 4), athletes will have identified their major life needs, such as time with their family, and activities that bring gratification, such as playing a musical instrument. Additionally, via the development of emotional self-awareness, it is also possible to identify basic emotional needs, such as the need for respect. These needs are different from wants, though wants are often simply the result of an emotional need. For example, an athlete may want a new sports car, and while this want is clear, upon further investigation this want may be the result of his need to demonstrate his success, which may itself result from a deep feeling of insecurity. In this case, the athlete's real need is to develop self-confidence. Identifying the fundamental needs and putting strategies in place to allow these needs to be met is one of the most important emotional regeneration strategies available.

Utilize effective goals and feedback.

The need for effective goals and feedback was stressed in Pillar 1 (refer to Chapter 4). This issue has a massive impact on the effectiveness of emotional recovery. The achievement of goals, together with feelings of moving forward and achievement, greatly enhances the feelings associated with optimal recovery states. This process is also linked with identifying activities that bring gratification, as outlined in Pillar 1. A mix of purely relaxing, pleasurable activities, together with activities that produce gratification, will greatly enhance an athlete's recovery potential.

Develop emotional regeneration strategies and have fun.

These strategies are again linked to the emotional quadrant. Over time, the athlete needs to identify activities that promote feelings associated with the low-energy, positive quarter of the quadrant. These activities will likely be very individualized and will often correlate with the basic emotional needs. For example, if spending time with family is an underlying emotional need, any time spent relaxing with family will likely develop these low-energy, positive feelings. Additionally, athletes need to ensure that they spend time having fun and engaging in enjoyable pleasurable activities that again foster the required emotions associated with recovery. When choosing activities, it is vital to note that it is not simply the activity that matters, but also how it is utilized. Attention and psychic energy have to be invested in the activity. Otherwise, it will be ineffective. For example, spending time conversing with friends will not be effective unless attention is totally devoted to the activity. When the athlete is able to concentrate and interact effectively with the opportunities provided by the activity, the result will be effective regeneration, which requires an order to the athlete's thoughts. Unless this state is achieved, the athlete will simply focus on whatever is problematic in his life at the time.

Whatever activities are chosen, the two keys of using these activities are as follows:

- Control
- Psychological disengagement

Control

An activity such as watching television may produce positive, low-energy quadrant thoughts, provided that the athlete is in control of the remote. Being forced to watch other peoples' programs can result in the complete opposite of what is intended.

Interestingly, much research suggests that TV is not a good relaxation strategy, and far better strategies exist that can develop emotional regeneration, such as listening to relaxing music and reading. These types of activities require more effective ordering of thoughts, and eventually become more athlete-controlled than activities such as watching TV, where programming is controlled by the networks.

Psychological Disengagement

Everyone has probably been in a situation in which he is performing an activity, but his mind is elsewhere, preoccupied with issues stemming from work, relationships, training, etc. In these instances, what are normally relaxing activities (e.g., a round of golf), can in fact turn into frustrating, stressful activities—again, the opposite of what was intended. Hopefully, athletes will have established rituals by which they devote time each week to the activities that bring them gratification. Additionally, to maximize gratification and emotional regeneration, it is important for the athlete to identify whether he is disengaged before undertaking the activity. If not, the athlete should perform the disengagement ritual outlined earlier in this chapter.

Athletes must use "my time" and keep this time sacrosanct.

In modern society, opportunities for quiet reflection are tough to find. However, having adequate personal time is one of the underlying principles of recovery. In Eastern cultures, activities such as meditation and tai chi are an important part of everyday life, giving people time in which to recover on a multidimensional basis.

While not all athletes will be comfortable with these types of activities, it is important that athletes devote some of their time to themselves. This time may involve simple activities such as reading or listening to music. What is important is that the activity promotes relaxation and becomes a primary ritual. This time should be written into diaries and should not be negotiated.

Whatever activity is chosen, an athlete should develop an appropriate ritual to maximize the effectiveness of this time. Csikszentmihalyi (2002) outlines the following ritual, which could be used by someone who wishes to use music to promote relaxation.

- Set aside a time, and ensure this time is not disturbed
- Deepen concentration by setting up a preactivity ritual, such as sitting in a favorite chair and dimming the lights.
- Plan the activity carefully, including the session goals and the music to be played.

While this specific ritual may not be ideal for all activities, it does demonstrate how emotional regeneration can be facilitated through effective planning.

Summary

- The Performance Lifestyle strategy involves building capacity as well as recovery activities.
- Capacity needs to be built in all domains.
- Building capacity should entail periods of high-intensity activity that complies with the universal training principles.
- Following capacity development, a period of regeneration and recovery is needed.
- Athletes need to develop their own strategies for regeneration in the physical, psychological, and emotional domains.
- Only by addressing all domains will optimal performance and recovery be achieved.
- The effectiveness of recovery strategies is individualized, and athletes need to develop their preferred strategies.
- Recovery needs to be related to the stressors encountered in terms of both the volume of stress and the exact nature of stress.

9

Pillar 6—Quality Nutrition

"Let food be thy medicine, thy medicine shall be thy food."
—Hippocrates

Quality nutrition is a crucial part of any recovery strategy, and therefore is a key pillar in the Performance Lifestyle. An important aspect of performance nutrition within a Performance Lifestyle is that it is not simply what an athlete eats and drinks before, during, and after training and games that counts. While this aspect is important, it is equally important to take an overall view of nutrition. The Performance Lifestyle approach to recovery is all about how an athlete manages the process of recovery all day, every day. In the quest for optimum performance and recovery, the quality of nutrition throughout the week will greatly affect overall performance and recovery, and this aspect is stressed just as much as pre-, during-, and post-training nutrition.

Nutritional Requirements for Peak Performance

Quality sports nutrition is all about the following:

- Ensuring that athletes get enough quality calories to refuel after performance.
- Ensuring that quality nutrients are provided to optimize all body functions, and that these nutrients are provided at regular intervals.
- Ensuring optimal levels of hydration throughout each day
- Ensuring that athletes eat in a way that ensures that blood sugar levels remain stable and do not fluctuate.
- Minimizing the quantity of energy-sapping foods

Daily Nutritional Requirements

Before looking at methods of constructing an effective Performance Lifestyle nutrition program, it is important to take a basic look at overall nutritional requirements for both performance and recovery. Basic nutritional requirements can be divided into two types: macronutrients and micronutrients.

Macronutrients, as their name suggests, are required in relatively large amounts in the body. Proteins, fats, and carbohydrates are the three macronutrients required for body functioning. The quantity of macronutrients needed will depend upon a combination of an athlete's basal metabolic rate and the amount of calories used in other activities, including training. Basal metabolic rate refers to the calories required daily to carry out the body's basic metabolic requirements, and represents the minimum daily caloric requirements for normal body functioning. For athletes, training and recovery requirements will add considerably to this total, which needs to be reflected in daily caloric intake.

In terms of the relative quantities of macronutrients, the general requirements for health also apply to athletics. Ideally, athletes should be consuming calories according to the following general breakdown:

- Carbohydrates: 60 percent
- Protein: 20 percent
- Fats: 20 percent

This breakdown provides a rough framework for the intake of macronutrients. It is important to note than some variations may occur within these guidelines according to the type of training being undertaken. Strength athletes may require a slightly larger relative protein intake, while endurance athletes may require a higher proportion of carbohydrate.

However, even when these percentages are adhered to, this breakdown is not necessarily sufficient for optimum nutrition. Within the macronutrient percentages, general guidelines exist for the best choice of foods to provide the required calories within each group. When these guidelines are followed, the optimum benefit from the framework can be achieved.

Proteins

Proteins are made up of amino acids, the building blocks of both protein and muscle. While the body can produce some amino acids, it must take in the others through the diet. The amino acids it can produce are called nonessential amino acids, while the ones it cannot produce, which therefore need to be taken in via the diet, are called essential amino acids. Complete proteins contain all of the essential amino acids, while protein sources that are lacking in one or more essential amino acids are termed incomplete. Animal-based proteins are the best forms of protein, as they are complete. While vegetable-based protein sources are available, they are normally incomplete and therefore need to be combined with other sources to provide all of the essential amino acids.

While animal proteins are preferred, they often contain large quantities of what can be termed "bad" fats (covered later in this chapter). When choosing protein sources, athletes should look for sources low in saturated fat. Fish and chicken are two of the best sources of protein. Red meat, which often gets poor press, is useful in the diet, but should be consumed only two to three times per week and should always come from lean cuts. Eggs and low-fat dairy products are also good sources of protein. Figure 9-1 lists the preferred sources of proteins.

Guidelines for Choosing Proteins	
Best	Skinless chicken or turkey, non-fried fish, 95 percent lean ground beef, egg whites, fat-free milk, and yogurt (low-fat/low-sugar)
Neutral	Chicken or turkey with skin, 1 to 2 percent dairy products (milk, cottage cheese, yogurt), whole eggs, trimmed pork, lean turkey bacon, 85 percent lean ham, and 85 to 90 percent lean beef
Worst	Bacon, processed meats, fried chicken, fried fish, marbled beef, lamb, cheese, and whole-fat dairy products

Figure 9-1

In terms of quantities, the amount will depend upon the athlete's sport and training. If the sport and training are endurance-based, athletes should look to consume 1.2 grams of protein per kilogram of body weight. However, if the sport or training is strength-based, then the athletes require greater amounts of protein, with 1.6 gram per kilogram of body weight being advised. Additionally, a limit exists to how much protein can be assimilated at any one sitting. Therefore, the best way to take in protein is in smaller portions eaten more regularly, rather than large infrequent intakes. This change often requires a radical change in some strength athletes, who are used to massive portions of meat at sittings.

Carbohydrates

Carbohydrates are the body's preferred energy source for sports and are essential for performance. Low-carbohydrate diets are simply not an option for athletes wanting to optimize their performance and recovery. Carbohydrates can be classified according to a concept called the glycemic index (Figure 9-2). This tool gives an indication of how rapidly the carbohydrate is digested, leading to a rise in blood sugar. Sugar and sugar-based products (with a very high glycemic index), for example, are rapidly digested, and the sugars enter the bloodstream rapidly, raising the blood sugar level and providing a sugar rush. However, this scenario quickly leads to the secretion of insulin, the role of which is to regulate blood sugar. A rapid lowering of blood sugar soon follows and can kick off an energy trough and a craving for more sugar. This yo-yo effect is not conducive to performance or recovery, and the athlete should try to avoid it as much as possible.

Glycemic Index (GI) of Common Carbohydrates

	High GI	**Medium GI**	**Low GI**
Breads and grains	Bagels, baguettes, croissants, doughnuts, muffins, pancakes, white bread, granola bars, waffles	Whole-grain breads, pita bread	100 percent stone-ground whole-wheat bread, whole-grain high-fiber bread
Vegetables	Parsnips, jacket and mashed potatoes	New and boiled potatoes	Sweet potatoes, yams, asparagus, broccoli, sprouts, bell peppers, carrots, celery, mushrooms, tomatoes, cucumbers
Fruit	Sweetened fruit juices, canned fruits in syrup, melons, dried fruits	Dates	Apples, apricots, bananas, cherries, kiwi, mangoes, oranges, blackberries, strawberries, raspberries, peaches, plums, blueberries
Cereals	Sugar-coated varieties	Corn-based cereals, rice-based cereals, Shredded Wheat®	Regular oatmeal (not instant), All Bran®
Rice and pasta	White rice, instant rice, short-grain rice	Macaroni	Basmati rice, brown rice, most types of whole-wheat pasta
Legumes and beans	Tapioca		Baked beans (low sugar), butterbeans, black-eyed beans, lentils, soy beans

Figure 9-2

By consuming low-glycemic foods, the athlete slows digestion and the related sugar release, and the yo-yo effect does not occur—the ideal situation to achieve via nutrition. Therefore, whenever possible, athletes should choose moderate-to low-glycemic foods. If an athlete does feel like eating high-glycemic foods, he should eat them in small quantities and in conjunction with low-glycemic foods, which will lower the overall glycemic load (the overall glycemic effect of the meal). Also, by combining the food with fats and proteins, the speed of absorption can be reduced, reducing the overall glycemic load of the meal and reducing the yo-yo effect.

Fats

Fats receive a bad rap and are seen as something to avoid in the diet. The trend for low-fat foods is everywhere, with "low-fat" being touted as healthy, despite the fact that many of these "low-fat" products contain high levels of sugar and play havoc with blood sugar levels. An important concept to remember is that not all fats are bad, and some are positively good. All diets need a supply of these good fats.

Fats play an important role in bodily functions and energy production, and athletes need to ensure that they have appropriate supplies of essential fatty acids (EFA). Fats, in addition to being an energy source, provide for nutrients and antioxidants. Omega-3 and omega-6 fatty acids are the two key EFA, and every athlete should be proactive in including these fats in their diet. Both of these fats assist in mental clarity and general health through their antioxidant qualities, and need to be an integral part of a Performance Lifestyle diet. Sources of omega-3 and omega-6 fatty acids are presented in Figure 9-3.

Sources of Omega-3 and Omega-6 Fatty Acids	
Type	**Major Sources**
Omega-3	Grain products, meats, oils (safflower, sunflower)
Omega-6	Oily fish (salmon, mackerel, trout, herring, sardines), leafy green vegetables

Figure 9-3

What athletes need to avoid are trans-fatty acids and hydrogenated and "partially hydrogenated" fats. These fats have a very negative effect on health and performance and therefore can hinder effective recovery. A danger is that despite their labels, low-fat products will often contain these fats. Athletes need to learn to read labels and look out for these bad fats. Figure 9-4 outlines good fats and bad fats.

Guidelines for Fat Intake	
Best	Olive oil, fish oil, canola oil, flaxseed oil, sunflower seeds, and nuts (almonds, cashews, pecans, walnuts)
Neutral	Peanuts
Worst	Animal fats, butter, cream, whole milk, lard, and brazil nuts

Figure 9-4

Water

Hydration is vital for performance, and water can be thought of as the fourth key macronutrient. Anytime an athlete is dehydrated, his performance level and recovery decline. Even slight dehydration results in substantial performance reduction, and hydration rituals need to be a vital part of any performance nutrition program.

Unfortunately, many people are dehydrated and simply do not realize it. Thirst is a poor indicator of hydration levels, and being thirsty means that dehydration has already set in. Urine color can be a useful indicator of hydration level. Ideally, urine should be clear. Any time it gets darker, it indicates the need to drink–and water is the ideal drink.

Planning a Meal

A key to achieving the recommended proportions of nutrients is effectively planning meals. When planning or selecting a meal, the following guidelines can assist athletes in making good decisions:

- *Add color to the plate*: As a first step, an athlete should add some vegetables, fruit, or nuts to his plate and vary as much in terms of color as possible. Doing so will help ensure that many vitamins and minerals are provided. In general, the more different colors an athlete adds, the greater the variety of nutrients he provides.
- *Add a lean protein source*: The protein source should be approximately one-third of the size of the plate. The athlete needs to avoid the temptation to load up on meat, etc., as a limit exists to how much protein can be absorbed at a time.
- *Add carbohydrates according to activity level*: On days of heavy training, an increase in the intake of unrefined carbohydrates, such as pasta, rice, etc., is recommended. On days of lighter training, this quantity should be reduced.
- *Hydrate*: Athletes should be in the habit of drinking water regularly and with every meal.

Performance Lifestyle Nutrition

Athletes need to develop a structure of eating that allows for the optimization of performance and recovery. The Performance Lifestyle nutrition program is built around seven key rules, which provide a structure for creating a performance nutrition program. In this way, nutrition can be programmed to maximize both performance and recovery. The seven key rules are:

1. Eat regular small meals.
2. Always eat breakfast.
3. Ensure a regular intake of fresh fruit and vegetables.
4. Unrefined and fresh is best.
5. Drink water regularly.
6. Eat a performance meal prior to bed.
7. Use chrono-nutrition.

Rule 1: Eat regular small meals.

A starting point for a performance nutrition program requires that an athlete forgets the normal three meals a day, as an athlete needs to ingest food at regular intervals. Eating smaller meals every two or three hours, also called grazing, is by far the best way for athletes to take in calories. This pattern provides for regular nutrients and, combined with effective use of the glycemic index, helps maintain blood sugar at a stable point. It is important to remember that, at times of hunger, the body is likely to use its own proteins as a source of energy. As the body's proteins are stored in its muscles, an athlete clearly does not want to break down hard-earned muscle. Eating regularly will ensure any muscle breakdown is minimized, and will also contribute to effective energy release.

The meals should follow the meal-selection guidelines outlined earlier in this chapter. By following these guidelines, mental and physical performance can be maintained throughout the day, without the peaks and valleys likely when eating fewer, larger meals. Similarly, this meal plan removes the hunger pangs that can often lead to overeating or the need to snack on convenience foods. Ironically, eating small meals is better for both gaining and losing weight, the only difference being the quantity of food at each meal. It is important that protein is provided at each meal, as protein promotes an anabolic environment in the body, one that promotes muscle growth and repair, both of which are vital for improved performance and recovery.

Depending upon the athlete's schedule, it may not be possible to eat formal meals this regularly. In these cases, well-planned snacks or shakes are ideal. Whichever option is chosen, athletes need to ensure that they take in the nutrients required at each meal.

Rule 2: Always eat breakfast.

Breakfast is often described as the most important meal of the day. Breakfast follows the longest period without food—overnight. It is vital that the athlete can provide the body with the nutrients required for performance first thing in the morning. A good breakfast is vital and should be a part of all morning rituals. Breakfast should always follow the meal-selection guidelines, as it needs to provide quality carbohydrates, protein, good fats, and fiber, together with hydration.

Rule 3: Ensure a regular intake of fresh fruit and vegetables.

Vitamins and minerals play an important part in many bodily functions, including growth, repair, and energy transduction. An athlete's aim is maximal performance, not simply to get by, and this objective will only be achieved with an optimal nutritional plan. Therefore, it is vital that all body systems are working at peak efficiency, which is not possible if any nutritional shortages exist. Fresh fruits and vegetables must be a part of any diet, as they are great sources of many of the vitamins and minerals required for optimal performance. As a rule of thumb, an athlete should try to include as many different colors as possible in meals and snacks—a simple way of ensuring that the widest range of vitamins and minerals are provided. As a general rule, a minimum of five servings of fresh fruit and vegetables per day is recommended.

Rule 4: Unrefined and fresh is best.

A characteristic of much of the food processing over the past few decades had been the replacement of nonrefined foods with refined ones. White breads, refined sugar, etc., are examples of this process. A general rule of thumb for athletes is to choose nonrefined foods whenever possible. In this way, they can control their blood sugar, while also maximizing the amount of dietary fiber consumed and the nutritional value of their food. When possible, fresh products should be used, again maximising the nutritional value to be gained from the diet.

Rule 5: Drink water regularly.

Dehydration has a serious effect on performance, which can occur at even low levels of dehydration. Similarly, dehydration can also negatively affect recovery ability. The amount of water needed daily will vary depending upon the athlete's size, his activity levels (both in and away from training), the environmental conditions he trains and lives in, and his clothing. For this reason, exact quantities of water cannot be accurately prescribed, and athletes should monitor their urine color to help them identify their levels of hydration (urine should be as clear as possible). However, it is not uncommon for male athletes to need to drink at least one gallon of water per day, excluding water needed for activity, while female athletes can easily require 0.7 gallons per day, to remain optimally hydrated. For athletes training in hot and humid conditions, adequate hydration is especially vital for optimal recovery.

Athletes need to be encouraged to drink at regular intervals. Indeed, a sports bottle should be their constant companion. While other beverages can add to fluid intake, water is the preferred source, as many other beverages contain large quantities of sugar or caffeine, which can have negative effects on recovery activities. It must always be remembered that thirst is never a good indicator of when to drink, because whenever an athlete is thirsty, they are already dehydrated. For this reason, they should never get to a position where they are thirsty.

In rehydrating after exercise, the amount of water lost through sweat is a good indicator of how much water is needed just to rehydrate. Sweating rates will be affected by the training load (intensity and volume), the environmental conditions (heat, humidity, and wind speed), and the clothing worn. In general, research has found that, left to their own devices, the majority of athletes fail to take in sufficient water postexercise to rehydrate. For this reason, all athletes should be encouraged to consume a large quantity of water postexercise.

Rule 6: Eat a performance meal prior to bed.

Unlike most dietary guidelines, which advise that food should be avoided prior to bed, the Performance Lifestyle advises a well-planned meal prior to bedtime. Pillar 7 emphasizes the need for sleep, which is when many recovery processes take place (refer to Chapter 10). For these processes to be optimally effective, an optimal supply of nutrients must be involved in the recovery process. Without a performance meal, the body will need to go many hours without nutrients, which is counterproductive to effective recovery.

The pre-bedtime meal should consist of slow-releasing proteins, which will provide an extended period of amino-acid availability, together with the positive nitrogen balance required for the body's anabolic processes. Casein-based supplements are useful at this time. This meal should also provide some unrefined low-glycemic carbohydrates that will provide for a slow release of carbohydrates, vitamins, and minerals.

Rule 7: Use Chrono-nutrition.

Chrono-nutrition refers to the timing of meals, especially in relation to training activities. In addition to eating well on a consistent basis, an athlete can undertake certain nutritional strategies around his training and competitions that can enhance both performance and recovery. What is important is that the athlete takes the overall guidelines and translates them into his own rituals. Any time that guidelines are provided regarding what to eat before, during, or after training or competition, they must always be tempered with the athlete's individual preferences, providing that the general rules are followed.

Precompetition Nutrition

The aim prior to competitions (or workouts) is to ensure that athletes have the required supply of the nutrients to power them through the competition and optimize performance. Ironically, by adhering to these guidelines, athletes are also able to optimize recovery by ensuring that they minimize the use of their nutrient stores. The guidelines also ensure that a supply of nutrients is immediately available to start the recovery process.

The key to precompetition nutrition is to match it to each athlete's preferences. How close to the competition does the athlete need to eat? Does he prefer liquid or solid food? It is essential to ensure that every athlete takes in the required nutrients, but never in a way that negatively affects performance. Athletes should avoid heavy proteins and fats that take a long time to digest and may lie in their stomachs during the competition or workout. Athletes should experiment during workouts to find out what works best, and then replicate what works during competitions.

Whatever they choose, athletes need to provide low- to moderate-glycemic carbohydrates and proteins, in a 4:1 carbohydrate to protein ratio. The protein provides the amino acids required for muscle growth and repair, while the carbohydrate is required to fuel and refuel the activity. Additionally, they need to take in a half-liter (0.13 gallons) of water. How long before the competition this water is taken will be a matter of preference, and athletes should experiment to find what works best for them. A useful start with the experiment is to work from two hours before a workout and evaluate how effective this method is. They can then adjust to a point where they feel their precompetition nutrition is at its most effective.

During-Competition Nutrition

This process can start once the warm-up begins and its aim will depend upon the type of activity. Overall, the main need is the replacement of fluids and electrolytes lost during the activity. The longer the activity, the greater the need for carbohydrates. Athletes can use carbohydrate drinks with a concentration of 4 to 8 percent, using medium- to high-glycemic carbohydrates. If the activity lasts longer than one hour, sodium and electrolytes should be added to the drink.

Postcompetition Nutrition

Recovery needs to start immediately after the activity, which is the one time when high-glycemic products are extremely useful. Again, what each athlete consumes will be a matter of his preferences, but he needs to ensure that whatever he decides to use is available immediately after the activity stops. Immediate intake takes advantage of a

Guidelines for Pre- and Postworkout Meals	
Timing	**Type of Intake**
Preworkout (two hours preworkout)	Low-glycemic index (GI) carbohydrate meal with medium- and low-GI foods) with a moderate amount of protein. Drink 500 mL of water two hours before exercise.
Immediately preworkout (<20 minutes)	Medium- and high-GI foods with a small amount of if needed protein; 4:1 carbohydrate-to-protein ratio
During game/workout	Medium- and high-GI sport product with a small amount of protein. Drink as much fluid as possible and replace electrolytes during longer sessions, or during sessions in high heat or humidity.
Immediately postworkout (within five minutes)	High-GI carbohydrates and protein using a 4:1 carbohydrate-to-protein ratio. Try to consume 1.5 g of carbohydrate per kg of bodyweight
Postexercise follow-up (within an hour)	Moderate- and high-GI carbohydrates and mixed meals with protein

Figure 9-5

window of opportunity during which the majority of carbohydrate calories consumed goes to replenish energy stores. As time progresses, this window closes until approximately two hours after training, when it shuts completely. To optimize recovery, athletes should make a recovery snack or drink part of their postcompetition ritual. This snack also needs to contain protein, again in a 4:1 ratio, to provide the amino acids needed to start the growth and repair process. When supplements are used, a mixed whey and casein protein is preferred at this time, as the whey provides for faster absorption and the casein enables protein intake to be delivered for a longer period.

The nutrition advice presented in this section is summarized in Figure 9-5. Athletes should use this information to come up with their own nutritional rituals that they can use before games/workouts, during games/workouts, and after games/workouts. In this way, their individualized Performance Lifestyle nutrition package can be developed.

Summary

- Quality nutrition provides athletes with the essential nutrients for optimum performance and recovery.
- Athletes need to aim for quality nutrition at all times, not only at workout/game time.
- Within the main food classifications—proteins, carbohydrates, and fats—great variations exist in the nature of foods, and athletes need to follow guidelines when choosing foods in each category.
- Meal selection needs to adhere to the four main rules to ensure optimal levels of macro- and micronutrients.
- The seven golden rules of nutrition allow an athlete to develop an effective performance nutrition program.

10

Pillar 7—Quality Sleep

"Sleep that knits up the ravelled sleeve of care,
The death of each day's life, sore labours bath,
Balm of hurt minds, great nature's second course,
Chief nourisher in life's feast."
—William Shakespeare, in Macbeth

Sleep of sufficient quality and quantity is essential for optimal performance and recovery. No person is able to perform optimally, in any sphere, unless he adequately addresses his sleep requirements. Research consistently shows that a large percentage of the population are sleep deprived, and are therefore unable to reach their full potential. This situation is no different in athletics. Indeed, high school and college students are among the most sleep-deprived people in society. For student athletes, this problem is often exacerbated by practice schedules being added to normal student requirements.

Unfortunately, in today's 24/7 culture, sleep is seen as something that eats into productivity, and is not valued. This attitude is counterproductive, as many people are constantly underperforming simply due to sleep deprivation. Even the slightest amount of sleep deprivation will result in a detrimental affect on mood, general health, performance, and ultimately recovery. For optimal performance and recovery, sleep must be seen as a necessity and not a luxury. Athletes need to aim for a state in which they are actively alert during their waking hours. Just as training well and eating well are normally accepted by athletes, sleeping well must be given just as important a role. Overall recovery and productivity will be increased, resulting in enhanced performance. Sleep must be an integral and valued part of an overall Performance Lifestyle.

What Is Sleep?

Sleep was once considered a passive, uniform state. However, research has shown that it is instead a complex elaborate cycle of states that facilitates recovery from the day's exertions and preparation for the next day. Sleep has been shown to consist of a number of different forms, each of which occurs in a regular cycle. Sleep is an active process during which key physiological, neural, and psychological recovery processes take place, with each phase of the cycle playing an important role in this recovery. As such, sleep must be seen as essential to an athlete's recovery and performance.

The Sleep Cycle

Sleep occurs in cycles, with each cycle consisting of a number of distinct phases. As a person lies in bed after turning the light out, his mind is still active and brain and eye activity indicate that he is still awake. As he drifts toward sleep, the brainwaves slow down and take on regular patterns, indicating a relaxed, but still awake, state. This stage is termed the alpha stage of sleep.

After a short time in this state, the brainwaves and breathing rate start to slow as stage 1 sleep is begun. Muscles start to relax and the heart rate slows, and theta brain waves start to dominate (50 to 100 microvolt waves of four to eight cycles per second). This light sleep stage can last from less than a minute to 10 minutes.

As sleep progresses, stage 2 sleep begins. At this point, theta waves are mixed with sleep spindles (12 to 14 cycles-per-second waves) and K complex waves (single high-amplitude waves). These waves reflect a move to what experts consider real sleep, short bursts of brain activity take place within the more stable pattern of theta waves. Muscle relaxation is evident as movement stops and real sleep begins. This stage lasts from 10 to 20 minutes.

After stage 2, a person then enters stage 3 sleep, where delta waves (very low-frequency, high-voltage brain waves) start to appear. Soon, the theta waves will disappear and delta waves will dominate, indicating the start of stage 4 deep sleep.

After 30 to 40 minutes of deep sleep, the process reverses through stages 3 and 2. However, rather than enter stage 1, something different happens, as a person will enter a stage of sleep called the rapid eye movement (REM) stage.

Following REM sleep, the whole sleep cycle will repeat itself. This process occurs every 90 to 110 minutes until a person is awake. Over the course of the night, the relative period of time spent in each phase changes, as time spent in stages 3 and 4 decreases and time spent in stage 2 and REM sleep increases. Unfortunately, if a person is awoken at any time in the cycle, the whole cycle starts again when they get back to sleep. For example, if someone was woken from stage 3 sleep, he would start again in stage 1. This restart emphasizes the importance of a period of uninterrupted sleep. Hence, the quality of sleep is as important as the overall duration. A long period of uninterrupted sleep is essential to optimize the time spent in deep and REM sleep.

The Key Sleep Stages for Optimal Recovery

While all of the sleep cycles play some role in recovery, by far the two most important stages are deep sleep and REM sleep.

Deep Sleep

Delta waves are indicative of deep sleep, which is vital for physiological recovery. During this stage, muscle relaxation is complete and blood supply to the muscles is increased. Additionally, metabolic activity is at its lowest, allowing for optimal tissue growth and repair. At the same time, growth hormone release is at its greatest. These processes, taken together, allow for the restorative processes required for physiological recovery to take place, especially if the nutritional pillar of the Performance Lifestyle provides the raw materials needed for optimal recovery.

Deep sleep has been shown to increase in duration after intense exercise, emphasizing its importance to recovery. Deep sleep is at its greatest in the first few cycles and can disappear in later cycles.

REM Sleep

During REM sleep, the sympathetic nervous system is at its most active, and blood flow to the brain is at its greatest. At this time, the eyes dart back and forth, despite being closed, giving the stage its name. It is at this stage that dreams are at their most common and their most vivid. During REM sleep, muscles are completely relaxed, leaving a person unable to move. REM sleep is essential for optimal brain functioning and contributes to psychological and emotional recovery. Additionally, it contributes to physical recovery, but on a neural rather than physiological level, with the replenishment of neural transmitters, the chemical messengers that allow neurons to communicate, a key factor. Without REM sleep, the ability to function on a physical, psychological, and emotional level is compromised. As the greatest amount of REM sleep comes in the later cycles, a continuous period of uninterrupted sleep is essential for optimal functioning in these areas. REM sleep is important at all times, but is especially important during periods when high neural stressors are present, such as during skill development or periods of high-intensity exercise such as power training. This need for REM sleep for brain function is ironic, as so many students stay up all night preparing for exams, while in reality their lack of sleep is ensuring that learning is retarded and that their brain functioning is severely reduced due to sleep deprivation.

Sleep Deprivation

Sleep deprivation affects a huge percentage of the population. Millions of people are simply not achieving maximal performance and productivity due to their lack of quality sleep. This statement is as true in athletics as in any other field. While people may focus on sleep deprivation after late nights or sleepless nights, sleep deprivation is as likely to occur over time as it is from single events.

Sleep deprivation is cumulative. An hour less sleep than required each day can lead to a cumulative sleep deprivation of seven hours over a week, the equivalent of a missed night of sleep every week. Carried on over a year, or indeed over many years, this situation leaves a person in a state of constant sleep deprivation—and a huge distance from optimal performance.

Another key fact to remember about sleep deprivation is that it does not dissipate by itself. Athletes who are sleep deprived need to act and make quality and quantity of sleep a key part of their Performance Lifestyles. Sleep deprivation is clearly a major problem. How do you know whether your athletes are sleep deprived? Figure 10-1 is designed to help athletes identify whether or not they are sleep deprived. If athletes have a score of 3 or more in any two of more of these questions, it could indicate a sleep-deprived state. The more 3s present, the more likely it is that the athlete is sleep deprived.

Performance Lifestyle—Sleep

Dr. James Maas (2001) outlines four golden rules of sleep. These golden rules need to become the framework around which an athlete builds his Performance Lifestyle sleep pillar:

- Get an adequate amount of sleep every day.
- Establish a regular sleep schedule.
- Get continuous sleep.
- Pay back lost sleep.

Get an adequate amount of sleep every day.

Sleep can be seen as a bank account. Each time a person sleeps he makes a deposit, and each time he misses a part of his required sleep he makes a withdrawal. As with

Sleep Deprivation Scale											
	The Scale										
I wake naturally.	10	9	8	7	6	5	4	3	2	1	I never wake naturally.
It's never a struggle to get out of bed	10	9	8	7	6	5	4	3	2	1	Its always a struggle to get out of bed.
I wake refreshed and energized.	10	9	8	7	6	5	4	3	2	1	I feel sluggish and tired when I wake.
I feel mentally alert, sharp, and focused.	10	9	8	7	6	5	4	3	2	1	I feel mentally slow and lack focus.
I never feel drowsy while. driving.	10	9	8	7	6	5	4	3	2	1	I often feel drowsy while driving.
Even boring activities do not send me to sleep.	10	9	8	7	6	5	4	3	2	1	I often fall asleep during boring activities.
I take about 20 minutes get to sleep.	10	9	8	7	6	5	4	3	2	1	I fall asleep as soon as my to head hits the pillow.
I never fall asleep while watching TV.	10	9	8	7	6	5	4	3	2	1	I often fall asleep while watching TV.
I don't feel the need to catch up on sleep.	10	9	8	7	6	5	4	3	2	1	I always feel the need to sleep in on weekends.

Figure 10-1

a normal bank account, it is important to keep the account in the positive (i.e., with more deposits than withdrawals). An adequate amount of daily sleep is a cornerstone of the Performance Lifestyle.

Establish a regular sleep schedule.

Pillar 4 established the importance of rituals (refer to Chapter 7). Rituals allow effective lifestyle changes to be made in the most energy-efficient way. A regular sleep ritual will involve going to bed and waking at the same time each day and establishing a presleep ritual (covered in greater detail later in this chapter).

Get continuous sleep.

Unlike nutrition, where the advice is for "little and often," sleep is best in continuous stretches. This pattern allows for the engagement of an optimum number of sleep cycles, thereby maximizing recovery. If this scenario is not possible, sleep should be supplemented by power naps (as discussed later in this chapter).

Pay back lost sleep.

Any time sleep is lost, it needs to be repaid or the account will be overdrawn. Any time sleep is lost, an athlete should try to pay it back using the suggestions outlined later in the chapter.

Optimizing Sleep

Within this framework, activities and rituals can be used by an athlete to optimize the quality and quantity of sleep. The Performance Lifestyle approach to optimizing sleep involves three main elements:

- Establish sleep needs.
- Establish strategies and rituals for optimizing sleep.
- Establish strategies and rituals to cope with times of sleep deprivation.

Establish sleep needs.

While this is process must be individualized, the normal amount of sleep required for optimal performance will be between eight and 10 hours per night. The reality is that few people are getting anywhere near the sleep they require. Many people are simply not aware of their full capacity because of constant sleep deprivation. An athlete is seeking peak performance, which requires maximal recovery. Sleep is vital for recovery on a physical, emotional, and psychological level, and an athlete must maximize these elements and not focus on just "getting by."

Sleep requirements will vary with overall stress levels and associated recovery requirements. The harder the athlete is training, or the greater the overall stress levels he is facing, the more sleep he needs. This point is vital, as any time training levels or stress indicators increase, an athlete should respond immediately by increasing sleep. Figure 10-2 outlines a system for establishing sleep needs.

Establish strategies and rituals for optimizing sleep.

Sleep can be optimized in many different ways. The Performance Lifestyle provides two primary methods:

- Rituals
- Environment

Presleep Rituals

Rituals are key to establishing appropriate behaviors. In terms of sleep, rituals can help an athlete go to bed in a positive, disengaged state. While the rituals need to be individualized, they should include:

Evaluating Sleep Requirements

Write down the time you get up (which you can seldom change). ________
Count back eight hours from this time. ________
Go to bed a half hour before this time. ________
Continue this pattern for a week.
Record how you feel the next day.

____
____
____
____

Do your indicators still reveal sleep deprivation?

Yes ____________ No ____________

If yes, for the following week go to bed a half hour earlier

Repeat the process until you reach a sleep time that removes the indicators of sleep deprivation.

Figure 10-2

- Relaxing activities prior to bed (refer to Chapter 8)
- Disengaging activities if needed (refer to Chapter 8)
- An appropriate night-time performance meal

The key to all of these rituals is that when the athlete goes to bed he is in a relaxed state, disengaged from the day's activities. The psychological and emotional recovery activities outlined in Pillar 5 (refer to Chapter 8) can be used as presleep rituals, as they are designed to achieve the same psychological and emotional states required for good sleep.

Humans are creatures of habit—hence the importance of rituals in the Performance Lifestyle. An additional factor in sleep is an athlete's body clock, which requires regularity. People respond best when they have a regular time of going to bed and waking. Once individual sleep requirements have been established, athletes need to set up times of going to bed and waking that ensure that they get this sleep every day.

The bedroom itself needs to be associated with sleep and be a place for relaxing. Prior to sleep, an athlete should undertake activities that involve relaxation. What this process entails will be a matter of individual preference, but could involve reading or listening to relaxing music. The important thing is the development of an appropriate ritual, and that these activities become associated with sleep.

To keep the body clock on target, an athlete should try not to change his waking time. Even on weekends, he should try to keep to the same waking time. If he does like to sleep in on weekends, he should ensure that he wakes no longer than an hour after his normal waking time. When he tries to catch up on lost sleep, he should do so by going to bed earlier rather than waking later. Similarly, he should try to condition himself to waking at the same time without the need for an alarm clock.

Sleep Environment

The bedroom should be a place in which it is easy to go to sleep. The environment in the bedroom can greatly affect sleep, both in terms of quantity and quality. The main elements of the environment are noise; light; temperature and humidity; the bed, mattress, and pillows; the décor; security; and the clock.

• Noise

Noise can obviously affect sleep. The reality of noise is that many times it comes down to what an individual is used to. Someone who lives in a city is likely to be accustomed to city noise, and thus be far less affected by it than someone who moves to the city from the countryside. However, not withstanding these factors, certain factors must be considered:

✓Sudden noises are more disturbing than continuous noise.

✓Low-level consistent sounds are less problematic than high-level noises.

An athlete can do a number of things to optimize noise levels. Sounds should be eliminated when possible. However, some level of noise will always be present that cannot be controlled. In these cases, athletes should try to sleep in rooms where noise levels are reduced (e.g., away from a main road). Alternatively, if noise does keep an athlete awake, he could use earplugs as an extra form of defense. Earplugs can be a great tool for athletes on the road, where it is difficult to predetermine noise levels, and can be included in the traveling athlete's travel bag..

• Light

The general advice is "the darker the better." Historically, sleep/wake cycles were affected by light. In modern society, these natural cycles are being eroded by the ubiquity of artificial light. Sleep is facilitated by darkness and athletes need to make their bedrooms as dark as possible. Quality hotels use screens and heavy curtains to create darkness, and athletes need to consider similar measures if their bedrooms are light and they are having sleep problems.

• Temperature and Humidity

Everyone has had nights where the temperature is high and they have had a disturbed and uncomfortable night's sleep. People sleep best at approximately 65° F (18° C). Extreme temperatures, both high and low, can negatively affect sleep. Athletes should look for an environment where the temperature is controllable.

Body temperature can also be affected by what is worn to bed, either too much or too little. Clothing needs to be adjusted appropriately to achieve a situation in which the body is a degree or so warmer than the head.

Humidity is also a consideration. An ideal relative humidity is between 60 and 70 percent. The use of humidifiers or dehumidifiers can assist in achieving this level of humidity.

• The Bed, Mattress, and Pillows

The bed, including the mattress and pillows, will have a great affect on sleep. Ideally, an athlete should look for a bed that is as big as possible and at least six inches longer than he is.

A quality mattress is another important consideration. A mattress should provide for both support and a comfortable night's sleep. If the mattress is old, worn, or is no longer providing a suitable amount of support, then it may be time to get a new one. The mattress should provide comfortable support at all points of the body. An athlete should go to a quality store and try a good brand, and then assess whether his current mattress matches up. A good mattress is an excellent investment for the Performance Lifestyle, in that it enhances the quality of sleep and the level of recovery.

Good pillows that provide adjustability and can be molded into shape provide support where it is needed depending upon sleep position. Good pillows are a wise investment and, just like training gear, should be replaced when they cannot provide the appropriate support. A good pillow puts the head and spine in a mechanically efficient position and can contribute to reduced neck and back problems and enhanced sleep.

• The Décor

Room décor should be as tranquil as possible, with pale colors dominating. These colors are associated with peace and tranquillity. Athletes should avoid bright colors, as they will have the opposite effect. The bedroom should be clean and free from clutter to promote a peaceful environment.

- Security

While security may at first seem a strange consideration, people are more likely to sleep soundly if they feel safe. Therefore, effective door locks, etc., that create a safe environment are important. An athlete does not want to be in a situation where any time he hears a noise his mind starts racing because of a lack of security in the home.

- The Clock

How many times have you lied awake, glancing at the bright display of the clock? As you continue to be unable to sleep, the clock is staring back at you. You start counting each minute, with your mind slowly being taken over by the time. An athlete should try to avoid this situation by ensuring that any clocks he uses do not dominate the room and result in this type of situation. If he does use this type of clock, he should have it face away from him.

Strategies for Dealing With Sleep Deprivation

The first aspect of dealing with sleep deprivation is to acknowledge that sleep is a vital part of performance and that any lack of sleep needs to be caught up on. Ideally, an athlete should try to get an adequate amount of quality sleep each night, as doing so is the key to this pillar of the Performance Lifestyle. Missing sleep and then trying to catch up is not an effective long-term strategy. However, times will arise when an athlete is unable to get the required quantity of sleep. In these situations, he needs strategies to deal with the problem. In terms of the bank account outlined earlier, athletes should ensure that any time they make a withdrawal, they pay back what they withdrew.

Pay back the debt gradually.

While a common approach to catching up on sleep is to sleep in on weekends, it is important to remember that the body does not operate a different body clock for weekends. When athletes try to catch up on sleep, they should try to keep their waking time roughly the same (no more than an hour later), and try to go to bed slightly earlier. Going to bed earlier on the days following lost sleep is greatly preferred to later waking times, as it does not disrupt the body clock to anywhere near the same degree.

Use power naps.

Power naps, short sleeps during the day, are great tools in the Performance Lifestyle. Indeed, they can be used at all times, whether or not the athlete is sleep deprived, and can be used to make deposits into the sleep account. Power naps actually fit in with daily biorhythms, especially when taken in early afternoon, when the body often enters an afternoon trough. Power naps have been proven to provide some great benefits to mental performance.

Two types of naps exist, and their use will depend upon the athlete's particular requirements. The first is the normal power nap, which is roughly 20 minutes long and provides for an energizing, relaxing break from the day's toils. These naps are best taken in the early afternoon and, if appropriate, can become a regular part of the sleep schedule.

The second type of nap is much longer and is used to pay back a larger sleep debt. As these naps require a full sleep cycle, they need to last at least 90 minutes, and usually last two to three hours. These naps should not be regular occurrences and instead should be used in circumstances when a large amount of sleep needs to be repaid. Figure 10-3 provides guidelines for effective power naps.

Guidelines for Power Naps

- Find an environment in which you won't be disturbed and where you can relax.
- Switch off phones, faxes, etc., and put a "do not disturb" sign outside if necessary.
- If you can lie down, that is ideal. If not, use furniture that will give you the most relaxing position.
- You may want to set an alarm for 20 minutes later if you feel that you won't wake up.
- Carry out your relaxation strategy and try to sleep.
- Make this nap a daily ritual.

As with all rituals, this ritual will take time before you are comfortable with it. If at first you can't sleep, don't worry—just enjoy the relaxation. As this scenario becomes a ritual, you will find that your ability to sleep improves, and that the benefit you gain similarly improves.

Figure 10-3

Use prophylactic naps/sleep.

When a time of sleep deprivation is likely, naps and extra sleep can be used to guard against it. For example, when the travel schedule means that an athlete will lose sleep after a road game, sleep deprivation can be guarded against by getting extra sleep during the week leading up to the game. In this way, the detrimental effects of the loss of sleep will be guarded against by depositing sleep in the account to prepay this debt.

Strategies for Coping With Sleep Difficulty

Times will arise when, for whatever reason, an athlete simple cannot get off to sleep. Figure 10-4 provides strategies to deal with this problem.

Strategies for When You Can't Get to Sleep

- Don't try too hard. Instead, rather than thinking of sleeping, carry out a relaxation exercise in the bed.
- If this exercise doesn't work, get up. And if you know the cause of the sleeplessness, carry out your disengagement strategy.
- Engage in a relaxing activity. Pillar 5 will have given you an idea of what relaxing activities you could use. Try to avoid bright lights or stimulating activities.
- Return to bed when you feel relaxed and ready, but do not worry about the time or the consequences of the lack of sleep. You have strategies to deal with this problem.

Figure 10-4

If sleep problems persist over time, then the athlete needs to tackle the underlying problem. In many cases, the answers will be found in the preceding areas. While some cases will require medical assistance and may be the result of clinical conditions, many causes of sleeplessness can be solved. By asking themselves the following questions, athletes should be able to identify areas that may be resulting in a loss of sleep:

- Am I following a regular sleep schedule?
- Am I following a presleep ritual?
- Am I going to bed relaxed and disengaged?
- Am I avoiding stimulants or stimulating activities prior to bed?
- Am I getting up at the same time?
- Is the bedroom environment conducive to sleep?
- Is the bed conducive to quality sleep?

If the answer to any of these questions is "no," then the athlete may have hit upon an area to address. By following the guidelines associated with each statement, the athlete should be able to find a way to improve the quality of his sleep.

Summary

- Sleep is essential for both optimal performance and optimal recovery.
- The cyclical nature of sleep means that both the quantity and quality of sleep are vital.
- Deep sleep and REM sleep are the key phases for recovery.
- To optimize sleep, athletes should conform to the four golden rules: Get adequate sleep per night, establish a sleep schedule, get continuous sleep, and pay back lost sleep.
- Athletes need to optimize their sleep by establishing their needs, establishing rituals and environment for optimizing sleep, and establishing strategies to deal with sleep deprivation.

Bibliography

American College of Sports Medicine (1996). Position stand: Exercise and fluid replacement. *Medicine & Science in Sports & Exercise*, 28, 2130–2145.

American College of Sports Medicine, American Dietetic Association, and Dietitians of Canada (2000). Position stand: Nutrition and athletic performance. *Medicine & Science in Sports & Exercise*, 32, 12, 2130–2145.

Astrand, P.O. et al. (2003). *Textbook of Work Physiology*. Champaign, IL: Human Kinetics.

Baechle, T.R. & Earle, R.W. (2000). *Essentials of Strength Training and Conditioning* (2nd ed.). Champaign, IL: Human Kinetics.

Bompa, T.O. (1999). *Periodization*. Champaign IL: Human Kinetics.

Calder, A. (1996). Recovery: Revive, survive, and prosper. In: Gascoigne, H. (Ed.) *Smart Sport: The Ultimate Reference Manual for Sports People*. Canberra: RWM Publishing.

Covey, S.R. (1989). *The Seven Habits of Highly Effective People*. London: Simon and Schuster.

Covey, S.R. (2004). *The 8th Habit: From Effectiveness to Greatness*. New York: Free Press.

Csikszentmihalyi, M. (2002). *Flow: The Classic Work on How to Achieve Happiness*. London: Rider.

Faigenbaum, A.D., Mediate, P., & Rota, D. (2002). Sleep need in high school athletes. *Strength and Conditioning Journal*, 24, 4, 18–19.

Fleck, S.J. & Kraemer, W.J. (2004). *Designing Resistance Training Programs* (3rd ed.). Champaign, IL: Human Kinetics.

Goleman, D. (1995). *Emotional Intelligence*. London: Bloomsbury.

Hemmings, B. et al. (2000). Effects of massage on physiological restoration, perceived recovery, and repeated sports performance. *British Journal of Sports Medicine*, 34, 2, 109–114..

Heppell, M. (2004). *How to be Brilliant*. Harlow: Pearson.

Hewston, R.M. et al. (2005). The effectiveness of music as a strategy to regulate pre-competition mood. *Journal of Sport Sciences*, 23, 2, 181–182.

Hudson-Walters, P. (2004). Sleep, the athlete, and performance. *Strength and Conditioning Journal*, 24, 2, 17–24.

Jeffreys, I. (2004). A system for monitoring training stress and recovery in high school athletes. *Strength and Conditioning Journal*, 26, 3, 28–33.

Jeffreys, I. (2005). A multidimensional approach to enhancing recovery. *Strength and Conditioning Journal*, 5, 78–85

Jeffreys, I. (2006). Lifestyle monitoring in high school athletes. *Strength and Conditioning Journal*, 28, 3, 77–79.

Jeffreys, I. (2007). *Total Soccer Fitness*. Monterey, CA. Healthy Learning.

Kellman, M. (2002). *Enhancing Recovery, Preventing Underperformance in Athletes*. Champaign, IL: Human Kinetics.

Kellman, M. & Kallus, K.W. (2001). *Recovery Stress Questionnaire for Athletes: User Manual*. Champaign, IL: Human Kinetics.

Kennta, G. & Hassmen, P. (1998). Overtraining and recovery: A conceptual model. *Sports Medicine*, 26, 1–16.

Kubbitz, K.A. et al. (1996). The effects of acute and chronic exercise on sleep: A meta-analytical review. *Sports Medicine*, 21, 277–291.

Lane, K.N. & Wenger, H.A. (2004). Effect of selected recovery conditions on performance of repeated bouts of intermittent cycling separated by 24 hours. *Journal of Strength and Conditioning Research*, 18, 4, 855–860.

Loehr, J.E. (1994). *The New Toughness Training for Sports*. New York: Plume.

Loehr, J.E. & Schwartz, T. (2003). *The Power of Full Engagement*. New York: Free Press.

Maas, J.B. (2001). *Power Sleep*. New York: Quill.

Mack, G. (2001). *Mind Gym: An Athletes Guide to Inner Excellence*. New York: Contemporary.

Manore, M.M., Mason, M. & Skoog, I. (2004). Applying the concepts of glycemic index and glycemic loads to active individuals. *ACSM Health and Fitness Journal*, 8, 5, 21–23.

McKenna, P. (2004). *Change Your Life in 7 Days*. London: Bantam Press.

McKenna, P. (2006). *Instant Confidence*. London: Bantam Press.

Noble, B.J. & Robertson, R.J. (1996). *Perceived Exertion*. Champaign, IL: Human Kinetics.

Seligman, M.E. (2003). *Authentic Happiness*. London: Nicholas Brealey.

Seligman, M.E. (2006). *Learned Optimism: How to Change Your Mind and Your Life*. New York: Vintage.

Stevens, M. & Lane, A. (2000). Mood regulating strategies used by athletes. *Journal of Sport Sciences*, 18, 1, 58–59.

Tildus, P.M. (1997). Manual massage and recovery of muscle function following exercise: A literature review. *Journal of Orthopaedic and Sports Physical Therapy*, 25, 2, 107–112.

Tildus, P.M. & Shoemaker, J.K. (1995). Effleurage massage, muscle blood flow and long-term post-exercise strength recovery. *International Journal of Sports Medicine*, 16, 7, 478–483.

Verstegen, M. & Williams P. (2004). *Core Performance*. New York: Rodale.

Verstegen M. & Williams P. (2005). *Core Performance Essentials*. New York: Rodale.

Viru, A. (1995). *Adaptation in Sports Training*. Boca Raton, FL: CRC Press.

Viitasalo, J.T. et al. (1995). Warm underwater water jet massage improves recovery from intense physical exercise. *European Journal of Applied Physiology and Occupational Physiology*, 71, 5, 431–438.

Weinberg, R. S. & Gould, D. (1999). *Foundations of Sport and Exercise Psychology* (2nd ed.). Champaign, IL: Human Kinetics.

Wrisberg, C.A. & Johnson, M.S. (2002). Quality of life. In: Kellman, M. (Ed.) *Enhancing Recovery: Preventing Underperformance in Athletes*. Champaign, IL; Human Kinetics.

Zatsiorsky, V. (1995). *The Science and Practice of Strength Training*. Champaign, IL: Human Kinetics.

Ziegenfus, T. (2004). Post-workout carbohydrate and protein supplementation. *Strength and Conditioning Journal*, 26, 3, 43–44.

About the Author

Ian Jeffreys, B.A. (Hons), MSc, CSCS*D, NSCA-CPT, ASCC, PGCE, is a senior lecturer in strength and conditioning at the University of Glamorgan in Pontypridd, Wales, UKE where he is also the lead strength and conditioning coach. He is also the proprietor and performance director of All-Pro Performance in Brecon, Wales.

Jeffreys is one of the leading strength and conditioning coaches in the United Kingdom (UK) and acts as a consultant to a number of athletes and teams. He is a director of the United Kingdom Strength and Conditioning Association (UKSCA), an "Accredited Member" of the UKSCA, and an assessor for the UKSCA accreditation procedure. He is also a tutor for the UKSCA education program. Jeffreys is a British Olympic Association registered strength and conditioning professional and a UK Athletics Level 3 Performance Coach for Sprints. He directs the talented athlete program for the County of Powys and is also the strength and conditioning advisor to the Welsh Rugby Union National Squad at Under 16 level. Jeffreys is a former professional rugby player who played at the professional level for 15 years.

Jeffreys is a longstanding member of the National Strength and Conditioning Association (NSCA), where he is a Certified Strength and Conditioning Specialist, re-certified with Distinction (CSCS,*D). He is a NSCA Coach Practitioner, and also a Certified Personal Trainer (NSCA-CPT), re-certified with Distinction (NSCA-CPT*D). He was voted the NSCA High School Professional of the Year in 2006.

Jeffreys is the editor of the UKSCA Journal: *Professional Strength and Conditioning*, and is the author of *Total Soccer Fitness*. Jeffreys has authored a number of strength and conditioning articles that have been featured in international publications. He has also authored a number of book chapters in international publications, including the *Essentials of Strength Training and Conditioning*. He has also presented internationally on various aspects of strength and conditioning, including at both the NSCA National and Sport-Specific Conference.

Jeffreys lives in Brecon Mid Wales, in the United Kingdom, with his wife Catherine and son James.